Inguinal Hernia: Pathophysiology and Genesis of the Disease

Giuseppe Amato

Inguinal Hernia: Pathophysiology and Genesis of the Disease

Springer

Giuseppe Amato
Former Professor of Abdominal Wall and Hernia Surgery
Postgraduate School of General Surgery
University of Cagliari
Cagliari, Italy

ISBN 978-3-030-95223-5 ISBN 978-3-030-95224-2 (eBook)
https://doi.org/10.1007/978-3-030-95224-2

This Springer imprint is published by the registered company Springer Nature Switzerland AG
The registered company address is: Gewerbestrasse 11, 6330 Cham, Switzerland

Foreword

It was with great pleasure that I accepted to write this foreword to the book *Inguinal hernia: Pathophysiology and genesis of the disease* which my esteemed colleague Giuseppe Amato has conceived and is about to publish. The life of a university professor is studded with various types of scientific collaborations in different fields and above all with different people. Each offers interactive opportunities with exchanges that are certainly scientific but also human. But considering the many interactions I have had, those with Prof. Amato remain among the most appreciated and culturally dynamic. Several years ago, when for the first time my group of researchers from the Department of Pathological Anatomy and Histology of the University of Trieste received a proposal for scientific collaboration from Prof. Amato, I was intrigued by the subject of the research. But perhaps even more particularly relevant than the siren song was the joyful, fresh breeze of cultural novelty brought by Prof. Amato in his pleasant and sparkling way of proposing science. He displays all the enthusiasm of those who have studied a subject without getting tired of it, rather finding in its many layers that which is highly significant but concealed and which then scientific concreteness can be attributed to. Inguinal hernia is a widespread disease but on further studying this topic I realized that despite the high incidence, many aspects of this disease were still far from being defined. The long-term and fruitful collaboration with Prof. Amato resulted in a long series of studies aimed at highlighting the macro- and microscopic alterations present in the various components of the inguinal region affected by hernial protrusion. These results, obtained with a great spirit of self-denial and affectionate collaboration, were then the subject of specific scientific articles published in the most important journals in the field. The indisputable scientific value of our histological investigations performed on biopsies from patients and cadavers with hernia and compared to controls from cadavers without hernia has been proven by the numerous citations obtained from the published articles.

It also makes me very proud that, by combining our histological experience with the anatomical-surgical skills of Prof. Amato, for the first time ever, the histological mapping of the inguinal region affected by visceral protrusion was carried out. The scientific evidence found during these studies constitutes a milestone in scientific research and is of fundamental importance for the definition of the pathophysiology of the inguinal region. It is also with great satisfaction that I have become aware that our common investigative experience has served as the basis for developing the pathogenetical hypothesis on the origin of this multifaceted pathology so well described and documented in the book.

Although the exciting and productive professional relationship has left an indelible mark, documented with high-quality scientific production, I would like above all to emphasize the affectionate human relationship marked by sympathy and unconditioned esteem that have become intertwined in these years of mutual practice. These feelings, despite the number of years which have passed, have remained absolutely unchanged.

My sincere congratulations go to Prof. Amato for what he has been able to produce in all these years of career dedicated to scientific research and to the development of new therapy concepts in the field of abdominal wall pathologies. I am sure that the book that is about to be published will constitute a cornerstone in the knowledge of the pathology of inguinal hernias. My best and affectionate wishes go to Prof. Amato for a positive outcome of his dynamism.

Professor Emeritus of Pathological Anatomy and Histology Furio Silvestri
University of Trieste,
Trieste, Italy

Preface

In recent times, very few investigations have dealt with the pathophysiology of the inguinal area and the pathogenesis of inguinal protrusions, even if these interrelated subjects are crucial for understanding steps in the development of one of the most widespread diseases of all: inguinal hernia. My involvement in this topic started decades ago, as I disappointingly recognized how undervalued the specificities of this common disease were among the surgical community. At that time, I suddenly became aware that the way in which inguinal hernia is considered and managed was in evident contrast with the physiology of the groin. Then, my critical analysis went on as I made a simple reflection: are current methods of therapy coherent with the pathogenesis of inguinal hernia? I quickly realized that the treatment concepts were totally disconnected with the, at that time, still unaddressed genesis of protrusion and, really, interest in discerning the pathogenetic pathway of inguinal protrusions among experts in the field was very low. On the other hand, both in literature and during hernia congresses, the main theme of discussion concerned the frequent complications encountered after inguinal herniorrhaphy and its management. At this stage, an old aphorism, remembrance of my student times, enlightened my doubtful thoughts: how can we manage a disease without knowledge of its roots? In brief, the cure of a pathological event without etiological basis simply leads to empirical treatments which are a harbinger of mishaps and complications. This perception fully matched with the effective state of the art in the treatment of inguinal hernia: an abundance of unpleasant complications, unsatisfied patients and surgeons, a desperate search for a gold standard of cure. These are the typical features of an inadequate model of treatment which is unquestionably disconnected from the etiology. With these reflections in mind, I became more and more interested in this topic until my perspective of evaluating anatomical conditions encountered during inguinal hernia repair changed. Detailed photographic documentation during hernia repair procedures helped in corroborating updated understanding of surgical and functional anatomy of the groin thus improving the perception of macroscopic anatomical changes of the herniated groin. An additional, but significant, intuition characterized the following passage of the discovery: highlighting modifications of the microscopic structure in the inguinal area affected by hernia protrusion. I well remember how surprised I was on learning that in literature there was no reference concerning histological evidence of modifications occurring in the inguinal floor when a protrusion arises. This implied that decades of studies focused on the biochemical and ultrastructural changes occurring in hernia patients have been carried out without evidencing possible concomitant injuries of the inguinal components. In brief, ultrastructural, biochemical elements such as collagen chains, metalloproteinase enzymes, and similar have been studied in depth for years but the structure of the groin itself has not been investigated: a contradiction in terms! However, the link between these biochemical changes and hernia genesis had not yet been proven. This strengthened the belief that to clear the mists in this intriguing topic a study focused on detecting histological changes of the herniated inguinal floor was totally overdue. As a layperson in this field, I involved skilled histologists to collaborate in the research, that opened a previously undisclosed door and allowed revealing the physiopathological changes which occur in the inguinal backwall. This scientific experience constituted the first attempt ever of mapping the herniated inguinal area with a specific protocol. Degenerative changes of muscles, vessels, and nerves showing the typical trait of chronic compressive damage constituted some significant findings of the histological investigation. This collaboration represented an exciting experience for me that contributed to extending my skills from simple surgical practice to a more complete awareness of the intricate physiological phenomena regulating the metabolic events of each single tissue element composing the groin. Continuing along this pathway, I turned my attention to a more precise definition of the functional alterations occurring in the inguinal floor in the presence of hernial protrusions. The opportunity arose when I again encountered a characteristic type of double ipsilateral hernia referred to as pantaloon hernia. Analysis of the photographic documentation of the septal arrangement that separates the two protrusions gave input to an interesting study. It allowed defining the separating tissue diaphragm between the two hernias, a previously unknown component of the inguinal backwall: the septum inguinalis. The evidence of this previously unidentified component of the groin led to the updating of old-fashioned concepts of functional anatomy of the groin, which dated back centuries ago. Nevertheless, more importantly, it was a crucial element for definitely addressing the pathogenesis of inguinal hernia. The macroscopic and histological changes evidenced in the septum inguinalis further confirm the degenerative roots of hernia protrusion, which, as highlighted in so many macro- and microphotographs, can be characterized as a degenerative disease caused by steady orthostatic visceral impact upon the groin. All new evidence concerning pathophysiology of the inguinal area and the revealed pathogenesis of inguinal hernia presented herewith should hopefully contribute to updating knowledge in the subject. I look forward to advanced concepts of cure being developed to improve treatment results of this intriguing disease.

Cagliari, Italy Giuseppe Amato

Acknowledgments

Over the years, a group of colleagues has lent a significant support to the scientific investigations that form the body of this book. Herewith I wish to thank them all one by one: Furio Silvestri, Rossana Bussani, Vito Rodolico, Roberto Puleio, Giorgio Romano, and Antonino Agrusa. Special thanks also to Giuseppina Ficile for the excellent work done in finalizing the drawings of the book.

Contents

1 Gross Anatomy of the Inguinal Region 1
1.1 Introduction 1
1.2 Abdominal Wall and Groin 1
1.3 Muscular and Myotendineal Structures of the Groin. 2
1.3.1 Muscle Rectus Abdominis 2
1.3.2 Muscle Pyramidalis 2
1.3.3 External Oblique Aponeurosis 2
1.3.4 External Oblique Muscle 4
1.3.5 Internal Oblique Muscle 5
1.3.6 Transversus Abdominis Muscle 6
1.4 Folds and Fossae of the Posterior Inguinal Area 7
1.5 The Inguinal Ligament. 8
1.6 The Myopectineal Orifice 9
1.7 Hesselbach's Triangle 9
1.8 The Transversalis Fascia 10
1.9 The Inguinal Canal. 10
1.10 The Internal Inguinal Ring or Inguinal Sphincter 10
1.11 The External Inguinal Ring 12
1.12 The Spermatic Cord. 12
1.13 Nerves of the Inguinal Area 13
References. 14

2 The Pelvis: Gender-Related Differences and Impact on Visceral Protrusion Disease. 15
2.1 Introduction 15
2.2 Anatomy of the Pelvis 16
2.3 Anatomical Differences of the Pelvis Bones between Male and Female 17

2.4 Significance of Gender-Related Anatomical Difference in the Development of Visceral Protrusions. 19
2.5 Effects of the Orthostatic Vector Forces upon the Lower Pelvic District 20
References. 21

3 **Physiology of the Inguinal Area** 23
3.1 Introduction 23
3.2 The Inguinal Sphincter. 23
3.3 Integrated Muscular Features of the Groin 24
References. 26

4 **Pathological Anatomy and Histology of the Herniated Groin** 29
4.1 Introduction 29
4.2 The Protocol of Histological Investigation in the Herniated Groin 30
4.3 Analysis of Histological Findings 31
4.4 Damage to Inguinal Vascular Structures and Related Implications 32
4.5 Structural Damage Occurring in the Nervous Network of the Inguinal District 35
4.6 Histological Evidence of Muscular Injuries in the Herniated Groin 36
4.7 Effects of the Histologically Evidenced Damage on the Physiology of Inguinal Structures. 40
4.8 Chronic Compression on the Inguinal Barrier Leading to Tissue Degeneration. Which Source? 41
References. 42

5 **The Septum Inguinalis: Its Role in the Pathogenesis of Inguinal Hernia**. 45
5.1 Introduction 45
5.2 Components of the Septum Inguinalis. 46
5.3 Gross Anatomical Modifications of Septum Inguinalis in the Herniated Groin 46
5.4 Histological Modification of Septum Inguinalis in the Herniated Groin 50
5.5 Significance of Macro and Microscopic Findings Encountered in the Septum Inguinalis. 53
5.6 Steady Orthostatic Visceral Impact Is Source of Inguinal Hernia Disease. 54
References. 57

6 New Aspects in the Functional Anatomy of the Groin 59
6.1 Introduction 59
6.2 Morphology of the Inguinal Floor 59
6.3 Hesselbach's Triangle: First Report in the Functional Anatomy of the Groin 61
6.4 Critical Evaluation of Hesselbach's Functional Anatomy Concept Related to Inguinal Structures 62
6.5 An Updated Concept of the Functional Anatomy of the Groin 63
References 64

7 Classification of Inguinal Hernias Based on Functional Anatomy of the Groin 67
7.1 Introduction 67
7.2 Critical Revision of Inguinal Hernia Classifications 68
7.3 Proposed Updated Classification Based on the Functional Anatomy of the Groin 68
7.3.1 Do we Need another Hernia Classification List? Let us Explain this New One 79
7.4 Accurate Intraoperative Classification of Inguinal Hernia May Improve Surgical Treatment Results 81
References 81

8 State of the Art and Future Perspectives in Inguinal Hernia Repair 83
8.1 State of the Art in the Treatment of Inguinal Hernia 83
8.2 Is Overcoming the Incongruences of the Currently Available Concept of Cure Possible? 84
8.3 A New Advanced Vision for the Treatment of Inguinal Hernia 85
8.4 A New Category of Devices for a more Physiologic and Pathogenetically Coherent Treatment of Inguinal Hernia 86
References 87

About the Author

Giuseppe Amato graduated in 1977 at the Faculty of Medicine of the University of Palermo (Italy). He was a resident of the Surgical Clinic of the University Policlinic in Palermo until 1978. Then moved to Germany where he worked, among others, at the Surgical Clinic of the Academic Hospital University Frankfurt in Hanau, and at the Thoracic and Cardiovascular Clinic of the Göttingen University. In 1984, he obtained his specialization in General Surgery at the Aerztekammer Münster. Since 1987, he has been senior surgical consultant in various medical institutions in Palermo and Rome (Italy). From 2006 until 2010 he has been professor at the Postgraduate School of General Surgery of the University of Palermo and from 2016 to 2020 he was professor of Abdominal Wall and Hernia Surgery at the Postgraduate School of General Surgery of the University of Cagliari. Prof. Amato has carried out experimental and research studies in pathophysiology and surgery of the abdominal wall leading to the development of new therapeutic strategies and devices. Among these, he conceived ProFlor, the first 3D dynamic responsive device for inguinal hernia repair and developed the related surgical technique. Thanks to its intrinsic dynamic behavior, ProFlor achieves a fully different, regenerative, biological response compared to conventional hernia meshes. He also developed an updated concept of implants for fixation-free treatment of ventral and incisional hernias: the tentacle mesh. This device, aside a fixation-free deployment, grants a wider overlap of the abdominal wall allowing for sharply reduced length of procedure and postoperative complications.

Prof. Amato is a member of many scientific societies, among which are the American College of Surgeons, the European Hernia Society, the Italian Society of Surgery, and the Italian Society of Endoscopic Surgery and New Technologies. Prof. Amato serves as editorial board member and reviewer of renowned scientific journals and is often invited as speaker in medical congresses in Europe, the USA, and Asia.

Chapter 1
Gross Anatomy of the Inguinal Region

1.1 Introduction

For centuries, the anatomy of the lower abdominal wall, and specifically the inguinal area, has constituted a subject of scientific investigations that with the recent development of new technologies constantly deserves updating. Many renowned scientists have left their imprint in defining and categorizing the structures composing the groin. Starting from the seventeenth century, and throughout the following epochs, anatomical studies carried out by the scientists Poupart, Henle, Hesselbach, Lytle, and Fruchaud became well known in this specific field of expertise and these scientists are universally celebrated as pioneers of medicine. At first glance, the anatomical composition of the inguinal region looks simple. Nevertheless, if deeper attention is given to this multifaceted region it becomes evident that there is a complex functionality deriving from the peculiarity of the neighboring structures. Dynamic features of the visceral content, trunk, and thigh significantly impact the anatomy and physiology of this area. Therefore, defining the gross anatomy of the lower inguinal wall, and more in detail the structure of the inguinal region is essential for understanding this complex part of the body.

1.2 Abdominal Wall and Groin

The abdominal wall is a robust muscular structure bilaterally covering the abdominal contents from the xiphoid bone along the costal margin down the flank and iliac bone as far as the pubic symphysis. It acts as a shield that protects the viscera from traumatic events, similar to the lid of a pressure cooker, regulating intra-abdominal pressure, taking part in significant physiological events such as coughing, vomiting,

G. Amato, *Inguinal Hernia: Pathophysiology and Genesis of the Disease*,
https://doi.org/10.1007/978-3-030-95224-2_1

and defecation. When needed, it contributes to implementing expiration by forceful dislodging the abdominal viscera cranially.

From external to internal, it is structurally composed of four layers: skin, superficial fascia, anterior and lateral musculature with related aponeuroses, with the parietal peritoneum being the most internal layer. Its lower portion forms the inguinal region, which possesses specific anatomical and physiological peculiarities.

The inguinal area is a complex structure of the lower abdominal wall, bilaterally composing a merging point of anatomical structures, vector forces, and motile targets. Being part of the abdominal wall, it is composed of muscles, ligaments, vessels, and nervous structures that confer the distinctive trait of a dynamic environment. Nevertheless, a specific peculiarity differentiates the inguinal area from the rest of the abdominal wall: it contains the anatomical tunnel of the inguinal canal that serves as a pathway for the spermatic cord in males or the round ligament of the uterus in females.

1.3 Muscular and Myotendineal Structures of the Groin

From the midline laterally, the myotendineal structures of the inguinal region are:

1.3.1 Muscle Rectus Abdominis

This is a long muscle, ranging cranially from the xiphoid process and costal cartilages to, distally, the pubic junction and pubic tuberculum. Innervated by thoracoabdominal nerves, it compresses abdominal contents and regulates bending movements of the trunk (Fig. 1.1).

1.3.2 Muscle Pyramidalis

This is a small triangular muscle positioned in the lowest midline of the abdominal wall running parallel to the linea alba until distal insertion in the pubic tubercle. It acts as tensor of the linea alba (Fig. 1.1).

1.3.3 External Oblique Aponeurosis

The fascia of the external oblique muscle (Fig. 1.2) is a thin but robust aponeurosis that fully wraps the anterolateral abdominal musculature. Its fibers, directed downward and medially, join those of the opposite external oblique aponeurosis in the

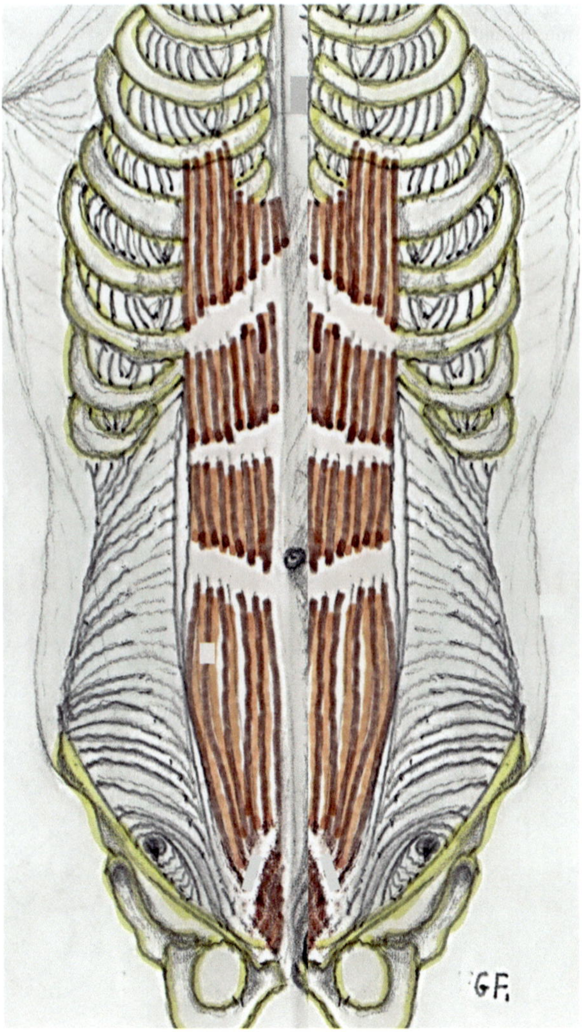

Fig. 1.1 Muscle rectus abdominis and pyramidalis © G. Ficile

midline forming the linea alba, which extends from the xiphoid bone to the pubic symphysis. Cranially, it is interconnected with the lowest bundles of the pectoralis major, while caudally it runs obliquely from the anterosuperior iliac crest to the pubic tubercle and the pectineal line forming the inguinal ligament. In the groin, from the anterior superior iliac crest and the pubic tubercle, the external oblique aponeurosis becomes evidently thicker, bending inwards giving rise to the inguinal ligament. In this configuration, it forms the roof of the inguinal canal, which is an anatomical tunnel that serves as a pathway for the spermatic cord in males. Closely above the pubic tubercle, the external oblique aponeurosis forms a wedge-shaped opening, the external inguinal ring, which allows the passage of the spermatic cord outside the abdominal wall, toward the scrotum.

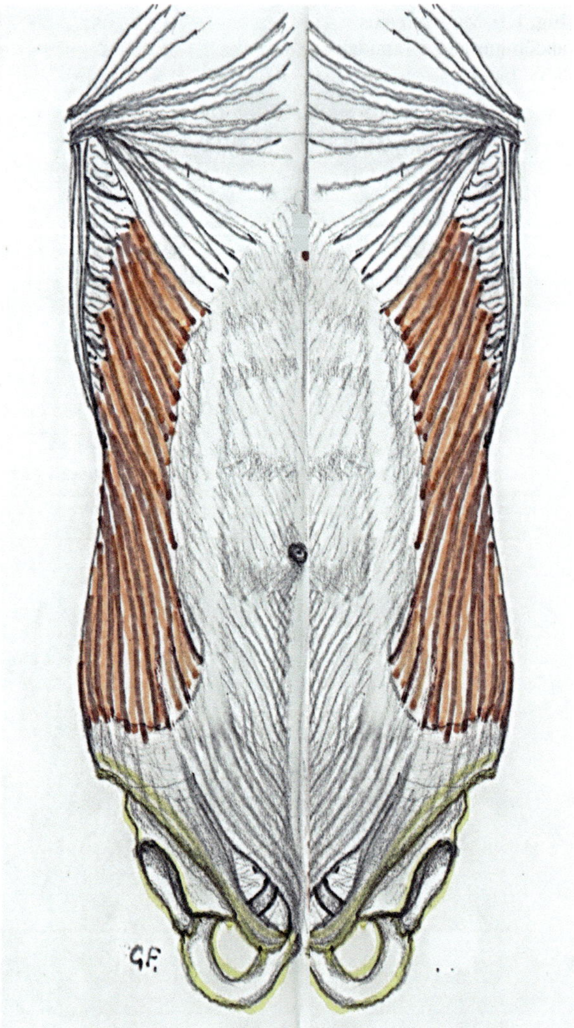

Fig. 1.2 External oblique muscle and aponeurosis © G. Ficile

1.3.4 External Oblique Muscle

The external oblique muscle (Fig. 1.2), originating from ribs 5–12, runs obliquely downward and inserts caudally into the anterior superior iliac spine (ASIS) and the pubic crest and medially to the anterior rectus sheath aponeurosis. It is considered the largest and most superficial flat muscle of the abdominal wall. Innervated by the anterior primary branches of T7-12 roots, it holds the abdominal wall and its contents, regulates intraabdominal pressure, helps in forcing respiratory movements and, cooperating with the external oblique of the opposite side, allows for rotation and abduction of the trunk.

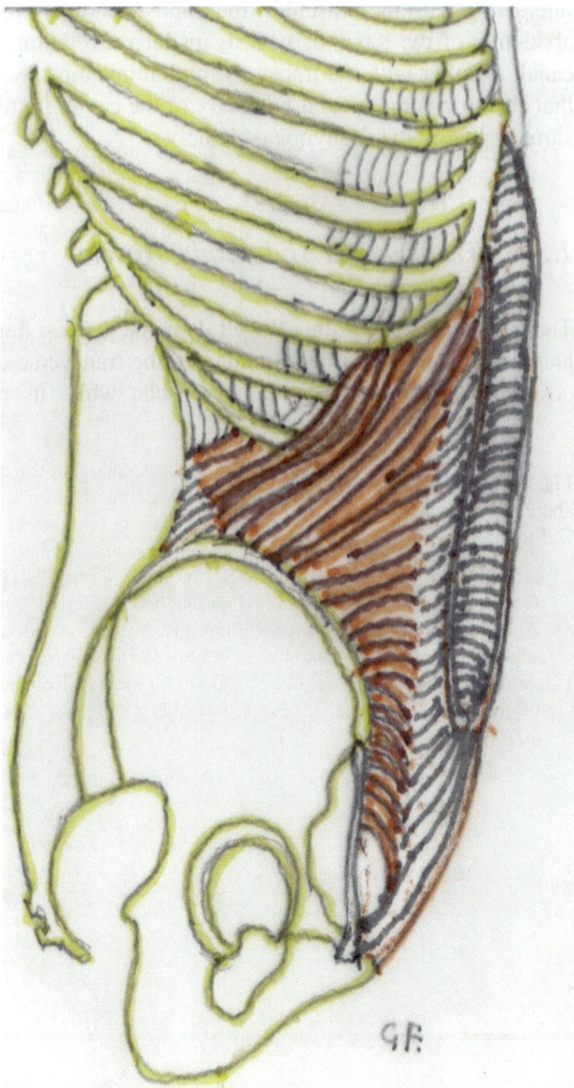

Fig. 1.3 Internal oblique muscle © G. Ficile

1.3.5 Internal Oblique Muscle

The internal oblique muscle (Fig. 1.3) is positioned immediately below the external oblique and, compared to it, seems less extended and thinner. Its fibers run in a cranio-medial sense (opposite to the external oblique bundles). Laterally, it originates from the lumbar fascia, inserts into the anterior half of the ASIS and runs medially downward to the inguinal ligament. Innervated by the anterior primary branches of T7–12 roots, it compresses the abdominal wall and its contents, modulates intraabdominal pressure, takes part in forced respiratory movements and, interacting with the muscle of the opposite side, allows unilateral contraction and abduction of the torso, as well as ipsilateral rotation of the trunk. In the inguinal canal, together with the transverse abdominis muscle, it forms the conjoint tendon that constitutes the medial boundary of the canal. In this area, it is often crossed or surmounted by the iliohypogastric nerve.

1.3.6 Transversus Abdominis Muscle

The transversus abdominis (Fig. 1.4) is the deepest flat muscle of the anterolateral abdominal wall with fibers running in the transverse direction. The top surface is covered by the internal oblique muscle, while its posterior surface is closely

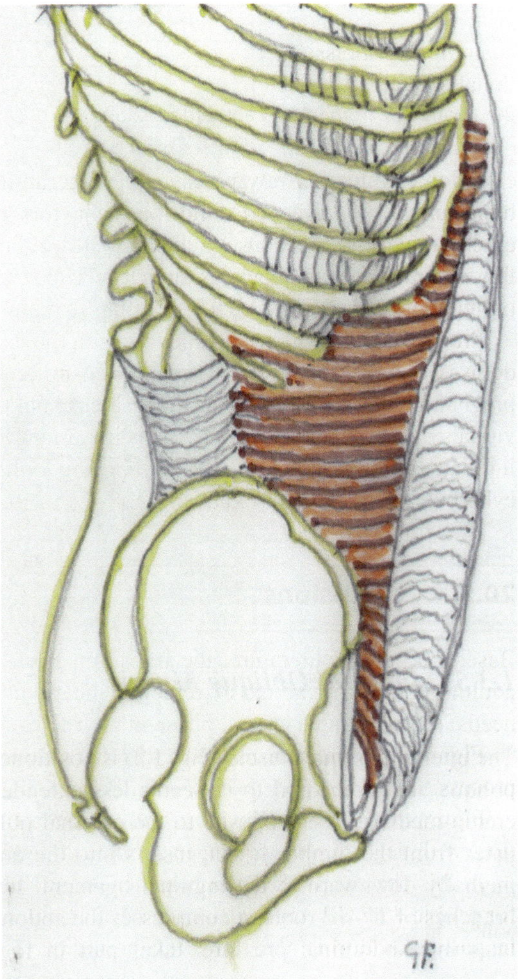

Fig. 1.4 Transversus abdominis muscle © G. Ficile

connected to the transversalis fascia. Cranially, it originates from the xiphoid process and costal cartilages 7–12; medially, it converges in the linea alba, laterally reaching the iliac crest and the thoracolumbar fascia, and caudally the pubic tubercle and inguinal ligament. Together with the internal oblique muscle, it forms the conjoint tendon which constitutes the cranial boundary of the inguinal canal. It is innervated by the thoracoabdominal nerves (T7-T11), subcostal nerve (T12), and branches of the lumbar plexus. Its functions include compression of the abdominal wall and abdominal viscera, regulation of intraabdominal pressure, and participation in forced respiratory movements.

1.4 Folds and Fossae of the Posterior Inguinal Area

There are three fossae in the lower posterior abdominal wall: the median or supravesical, the medial and the lateral, each bounded by distinct folds (Fig. 1.5). These anatomical depressions of the abdominal wall play a significant role in the functional anatomy of the groin since they represent the site where protrusions penetrate the myotendineal barrier of the groin toward the inguinal canal.

Starting from the median fossa, the urachus, a fibrotic structure residue of the embryonic ureter, is located on the preperitoneal surface of the abdominal wall. This represents the median umbilical fold, also called median umbilical ligament. The urachus is an unpaired fibrous remnant of the allantois, a canal that extends within the umbilical cord connecting the urinary bladder of the fetus and serves for draining fetal urine.

The supravesical inguinal fossa extends laterally to the urachus and is bounded by the medial umbilical ligament, remnant of fetal umbilical vessels. It forms a

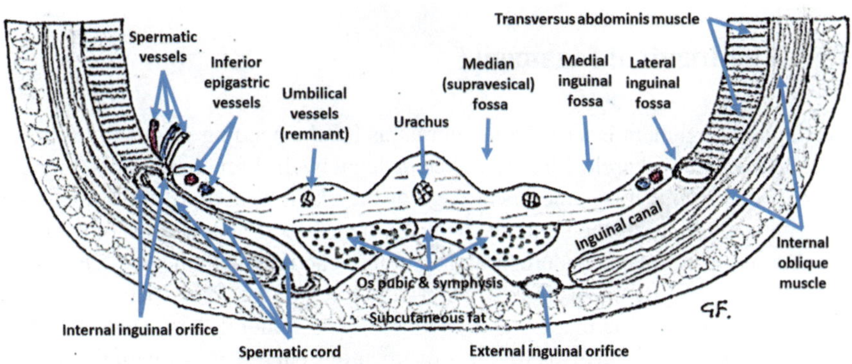

Fig. 1.5 Transverse section of the lower abdominal wall over the groin highlighting the inguinal orifices, muscular and vascular components, as well as fossae and folders of the posterior inguinal area © G. Ficile

relatively strong myotendineal barrier that under specific conditions can be penetrated by visceral protrusions. These hernias, referred to as supravesical inguinal hernia, crossing robust myotendineal structures such as the arcade of the lower rectus insertion to the pubic bone and the inguinal falx, do not always reach the anterior lying inguinal canal. Therefore, they remain within the structure of the abdominal wall, forming a non-exteriorized hernia: an internal supravesical hernia. This rare hernia type is usually diagnosed in emergency when visceral strangulation occurs. However, also the external type of the supravesical protrusion is characterized by a high rate of obstruction/strangulation of the herniated visceral content [1].

The medial umbilical ligament (cord of umbilical artery) is positioned laterally to the supravesical inguinal fossa, a paired structure running along the preperitoneal side of the abdominal wall. These obliterated vessels, remnants of the fetal period, are covered by the medial umbilical fold (plicae umbilicales mediales) that should not be mistaken for the median umbilical ligament mentioned above as a remnant of the embryonic urachus.

The medial inguinal fossa extends medially of the medial umbilical ligament. On the opposite site, the former is bounded by the lateral umbilical fold. This anatomical depression is the site where direct hernias arise.

The lateral umbilical fold, positioned medial to the deep inguinal ring on the posterior surface of the abdominal wall, envelops the inferior epigastric vessels: the artery (deriving from the external iliac artery) and its associated vein. Unlike the median and medial umbilical folds, the vascular content of the lateral umbilical fold remains patent and efficient after birth.

The lateral inguinal fossa lies laterally to the medial umbilical fold and the inferior epigastric vessels, its main structure is represented by the internal inguinal orifice, a sphincter-like structure that forms the internal opening of the inguinal canal. The lateral inguinal fossa, and specifically the internal inguinal ring, is the site where the most frequent inguinal protrusion arises: the indirect inguinal hernia.

1.5 The Inguinal Ligament

The inguinal ligament is a robust membranous band extending diagonally from the ASIS to the pubic tubercle. First described in detail by the French anatomist François Poupart in 1705, it forms the distal edge of the external oblique aponeurosis and constitutes the floor of the inguinal canal [2]. It is shaped by the fibers of the external abdominal oblique aponeurosis and continues caudally with the fascia lata of the thigh. Below this ligament, the muscular structures of the lower pelvis and thigh cross: the psoas major, iliacus, and pectineus. The femoral nerve and the lateral cutaneous nerve of thigh also cross this ligamentous band together with the femoral artery and vein, as well as the lymphatic vessel tributary of the leg.

1.6 The Myopectineal Orifice

The myopectineal orifice was first described by the French anatomist and surgeon Henri Fruchaud in 1956 [3]. It is bounded superiorly by the interconnected fibers of the transversus abdominis and internal oblique muscles, forming the conjoint tendon in the inguinal canal, and inferiorly by the pectineal line. It is divided by the inguinal ligament that divides this structure into two areas:

(a) The superior or suprainguinal area, that Fruchaud divided into lateral (site of indirect inguinal hernias) and medial (site of direct and supravesical inguinal hernias). However, this type of partition can be considered an anatomical limitation of Fruchaud's concept, as it does not consider the fact that in the inguinal area there are not two but three fossae: the lateral, the medial, and the supravesical. Therefore, a correct partition of the superior area of the myopectineal orifice should consider all three anatomical fossae.

(b) The inferior or subinguinal area, which despite appearing wide, is effectively smaller as it is closed off by the already described muscles, arteries, veins, and nerves crossing below the inguinal ligament. Only a small area close to the pubic symphysis remains patent: the femoral ring. This is the lowest weak point of the abdominal wall and is the site where femoral hernias can arise.

1.7 Hesselbach's Triangle

This anatomical triangle was defined by the German anatomist and surgeon Franz Kaspar Hesselbach in 1806 [4, 5]. It is medially bounded by the lateral border of the rectus abdominis sheath, and laterally by the inferior epigastric vessels and their membranous sheath. The inferior border runs along the inguinal ligament where, encountering the pubic crest, the apex of the triangle is located. This anatomical structure is well known and, throughout the centuries, has been the source of several studies that deal with the surgical treatment of inguinal hernias. It is also universally known for being the site of direct hernias. However, the significance of a crucial anatomical structure crossing the Hesselbach triangle does not seem to be considered as it should be. Actually, Hesselbach and the majority of the subsequently involved scientists seem to have undervalued the fact that this triangular area is crossed by the umbilical ligament which further divides the surface of the triangle into two parts: the medial fossa and the supravesical fossa. This anatomical subdivision, which includes the presence of an additional structure crossing this area, plays an important role in better defining the functional anatomy of the groin, since, not only do direct hernia protrude through Hesselbach's triangle, but also supravesical hernia, which constitute a neglected although insidious protrusion type often mistaken for direct hernias [1].

1.8 The Transversalis Fascia

The transversalis fascia is an aponeurotic structure that covers the posterior, preperitoneal surface of the transverse abdominal muscle. It is a part of the urogenital fascial layer that covers the entire abdominal wall and is in direct contact with the pelvic and iliac fasciae [6]. Its thickness may vary depending on the site of the covered abdominal wall. The insertion points are the iliac spine, between the insertion of the transversus abdominis and Iliacus muscles, in the posterior boundary of the inguinal ligament it is between the anterior superior iliac crest and the femoral vessels; it continues with the iliac fascia in this area. In the inguinal area, it inserts into the pubis and the pectineal line and is reinforced by fibers of the transversus abdominis muscle, forming a thick, robust fascial layer. It merges with the inguinal falx forming a strong myotendineal compound. It covers the testicular vessels when entering the internal inguinal ring forming the internal sheath of the spermatic cord in males or the round ligament of the uterus in females. Its thickness is clearly reduced as it nears the femoral vessels. Lying over these vascular structures it continues caudally to connect with the anterior layer of the femoral fascia.

1.9 The Inguinal Canal

The inguinal canal is a myotendineal channel crossing the abdominal wall in the inguinal region obliquely and infero-medially. It is approximately 4–5 cm in length, and positioned ca. 1.5 cm above the inguinal ligament, running parallel to the medial half of the ligament from the internal to the external inguinal ring. It contains the spermatic cord in males and the round ligament of the uterus in females, both covered by the fascia transversalis and running from the preperitoneal space to the outer opening of the canal.

1.10 The Internal Inguinal Ring or Inguinal Sphincter

The internal inguinal ring constitutes the internal, posterior opening of the inguinal canal. Oval shaped, it is positioned lateral to the inferior epigastric vessels, ca 1.5 cm cranial of the inguinal ligament. Cranially and laterally, it is circumscribed by the distal arched edge of the transversalis fascia. The size of the gap is larger in males than in females but may vary from subject to subject. Formed by interconnected muscular bundles of the internal oblique and transverse muscles, it wraps round the spermatic cord in males and the round ligament of the uterus in females (Fig. 1.6). This muscular arrangement converges around the spermatic cord/round ligament as a highly dynamic structure which forms a highly motile reactive barrier

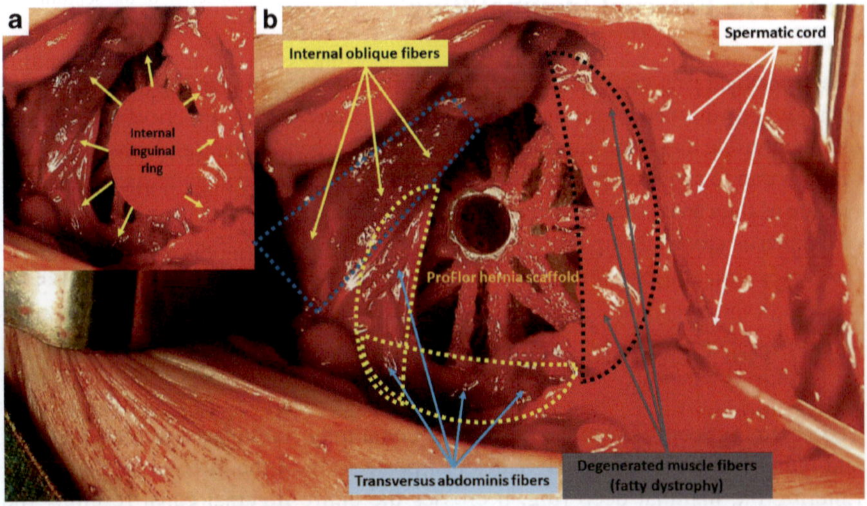

Fig. 1.6 (**a**) Internal inguinal ring highlighted after deployment of a 3D scaffold ProFlor during an inguinal hernia repair procedure. The centrifugal expansion of the 3D scaffold activates the sphincter-like contraction of the muscular arrangement to hold the device firmly lodged within the ring—(**b**) The intermittent colored geometrical figures highlight how the fibers of the internal oblique and transverse abdominis muscles are interconnected to compose the sphincter-like arrangement of the deep ring. This image also highlights a fatty dystrophy of the medial portion of the muscular structure forming the inguinal sphincter

to the increase of intra-abdominal pressure acting like a sphincter complex. Lytle [7] hypothesized the motile feature of this sphincter structure as an "inguinal sling" while Stoppa envisaged its motion as a shutter mechanism similar to a curtain closure [8]. However, the sphincter-like feature of the deep inguinal ring has recently been evidenced in vivo [9]. Considering that the most frequent inguinal hernia type, the indirect hernia, protrudes through this sphincter-like structure, it is not unreasonable to imagine that for some reason the contractile action of the inguinal sphincter becomes impaired. Following this line of thought, a series of histological investigations carried out in inguinal hernia patients demonstrated that, in these individuals, the muscular arrangement of the deep inguinal ring is affected, with significant degenerative damage of the muscle bundles outlining the ring seen in the form of hyaline degeneration from fibrosis to fatty dystrophy of the muscular elements. This structural damage was highlighted in a context of chronic inflammatory substrate composed of lympho-histiocytes and plasma cells [10]. Further confirmation of degenerative injury in this area arose from evidence of the involvement of the nervous structures, which showed typical signs of degenerative damage of the axons with fibrosis and sometimes Wallerian degeneration [11]. This multi-structural damage revealed the univocal feature of chronic compressive injury [12, 13]. Overall, this scientific evidence seems to confirm the hypothesis of the impairment of the sphincter-like action of the deep ring as the source of indirect inguinal hernia.

1.11 The External Inguinal Ring

The superficial ring constitutes the triangle shaped external opening of the inguinal canal. It is positioned cranio-laterally close to the pubic crest. Fibers of the external oblique muscle and intercrural fibers, which run perpendicular, reinforce this membranous gap to avoid widening the ring. In males, it is crossed by the spermatic cord outside of the canal which reaches the scrotum, while in females the round ligament of the uterus passes through it.

1.12 The Spermatic Cord

The spermatic cord is a tubular structure containing muscular, vascular, nervous, and lymphatic elements. It originates just posteriorly of the internal inguinal ring. Entering the inguinal deep ring, it crosses the entire inguinal canal reaching the external ring to enter the scrotal sac.

Ranging in diameter from 10 to 20 mm, it is enclosed by three layers of fasciae: the external spermatic fascia, the cremasteric fascia that contains the cremasteric muscle, and the internal spermatic fascia, an extension of the fascia transversalis. It encloses the vas deferens (ductus deferens), the plexus pampiniformis and the testicular vein. It is crossed by the testicular artery, the deferential artery and the cremasteric artery (Fig. 1.7). It contains the genital branch of the genitofemoral nerve, the ilioinguinal nerve and sympathetic nervous branches of the testicle. The

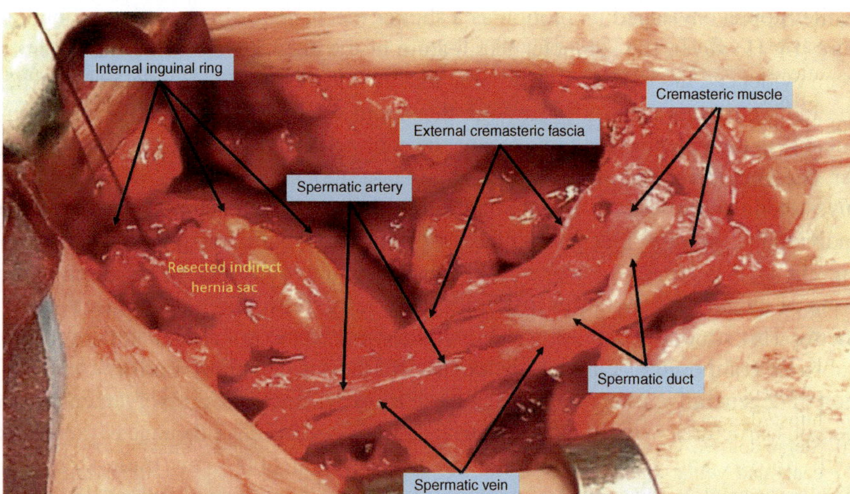

Fig. 1.7 Dissected spermatic cord in the frame of an indirect hernia repair after removal of the hernia sac. The opened cremasteric fasciae expose the spermatic artery, the spermatic vein, and the spermatic duct close to the fibers of the cremasteric muscle

lymphatic vessels ascending from the testicle and the tunica vaginalis (remains of the processus vaginalis) are also contained within the spermatic cord.

In place of the spermatic cord in males, in females, the round ligament of the uterus crosses the inguinal canal. It is a ca. 11 cm long fibro-muscular band originating from the cranio-lateral edge of the uterus, containing neurovascular elements. An intraabdominal path crosses the internal inguinal ring passing through the inguinal canal, which then exteriorizes in the subcutaneous tissue entering the mons pubis and the labia majora. It serves for the maintenance of physiological uterine anteflexion.

1.13 Nerves of the Inguinal Area

The iliohypogastric nerve originates from the cranial portion of the L1 spinal nerve. Running in the posterior surface of the latero-anterior abdominal wall, in proximity to the iliac spine it penetrates the transversus abdominis muscle passing through the interstitium between the transversus and the internal oblique muscle. In many cases, it remains bound between these two muscles but sometimes it penetrates the internal oblique and running above it the surface becomes visible in the inguinal canal (Fig. 1.8). Then, approx. 2 cm above the external inguinal ring it passes across the external oblique aponeurosis and, becoming subcutaneous, innervates the skin of the hypogastric area.

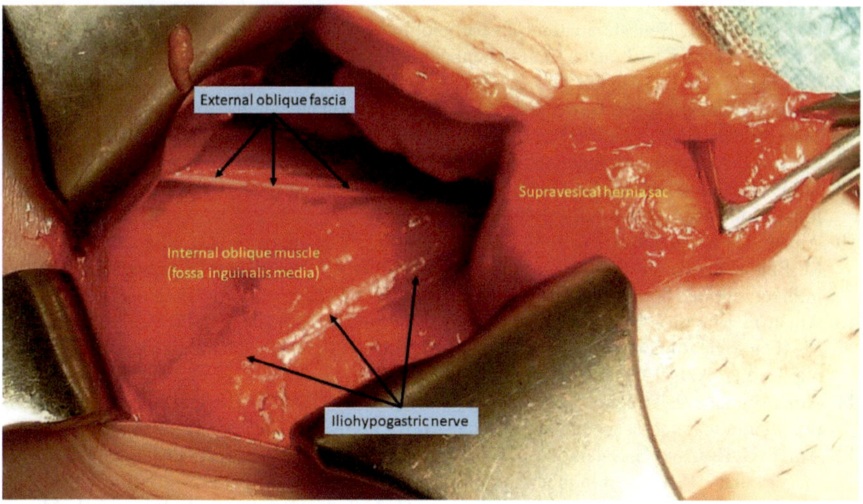

Fig. 1.8 The iliohypogastric nerve runs over the surface of the internal oblique muscle in the fossa inguinalis media. The image was taken during surgical treatment of a rare hernia of the supravesical fossa in a female patient

The ilioinguinal nerve is a ramus of the L1 lumbar nerve. From the lumbar region, it passes through the posterior surface of the lateral abdominal wall until it penetrates the transversus abdominis close to the ASIS in the inguinal area. Running between the transversus and the internal oblique muscles it often generates connections to the iliohypogastric nerve. Close to the inguinal canal it perforates the internal oblique muscle and continues its path lying over the superficial sheath of the spermatic cord, where in males it innervates the skin of the basis of the penis and proximal scrotal skin. In females, it runs over the round ligament to innervate the pubic skin and labia majora. Outside the external inguinal ring, it distributes its fibers to the skin of the proximal and medial surface of the thigh.

The genital branch of the genitofemoral nerve is a ramus of the genitofemoral nerve that originates from the cranial segments of the L1-2 branches. It runs inside the cremasteric fascia of the spermatic cord regulating the motile function of the cremaster muscle. Outside the inguinal canal, in males, it innervates the dartos muscle and the anterior scrotal skin, while in females, the pubic skin and the labia majora.

References

1. Amato G, Romano G, Erdas E, Medas F, Gordini L, Podda F, Calò P. External hernia of the supravesical fossa: rare or simply misidentified? Int J Surg. 2017;41:119–26.
2. Poupart F. Chirurgie complète. Paris, 1695.
3. Fruchaud H. Anatomic chirurgicale des hernies de l'aine. Paris: Doin; 1956.
4. Hesselbach FK. Anatomisch-chirurgische Abhandlung über den Ursprung der Leistenbrüche. Würzburg: Baumgärtner; 1806.
5. Hesselbach FK. Neueste anatomisch-pathologische Untersuchungen über den Ursprung und das Fortschreiten der Leisten- und Schenkelbrüche. Würzburg: Staheliano; 1814.
6. Li Y, Qin C, Yan L, Tong C, Qiu J, Zhao Y, Xiao Y, Wang X. Urogenital fascia anatomy study in the inguinal region of 10 formalin-fixed cadavers: new understanding for laparoscopic inguinal hernia repair. BMC Surg. 2021;21(1):295.
7. Lytle WJ. Anatomy and function in hernia repair. Proc R Soc Med. 1961;54:967–70.
8. Stoppa R. Como se forma una hernia inguinal? Actualizacion en chirugia del aparato digestivo. Fundacion MMA. 1984–2004;8:469–73.
9. Amato G, Sciacchitano T, Bell SG, Romano G, Cocchiara G, Lo Monte AI, Romano M. Sphincter-like motion following mechanical dilation of the internal inguinal ring during indirect inguinal hernia procedure. Hernia. 2009;13:67–72.
10. Amato G, Marasa L, Sciacchitano T, Bell SG, Romano G, Gioviale MC, Lo Monte AI, Romano M. Histological findings of the internal inguinal ring in patients having indirect inguinal hernia. Hernia. 2009;13:259–62.
11. Amato G, Ober E, Romano G, Salamone G, Agrusa A, Gulotta G, Bussani R. Nerve degeneration in inguinal hernia specimens. Hernia. 2011;15:53–8.
12. Amato G, Romano G, Salamone G, Agrusa A, Saladino VA, Silvestri F, Bussani R. Damage to the vascular structures in inguinal hernia specimens. Hernia. 2012;16:63–7.
13. Amato G, Agrusa A, Romano G, Salamone G, Gulotta G, Silvestri F, Bussani R. Muscle degeneration in inguinal hernia specimens. Hernia. 2012;16:327–31.

Chapter 2
The Pelvis: Gender-Related Differences and Impact on Visceral Protrusion Disease

2.1 Introduction

A common question asked of doctors by patients suffering from inguinal hernia concerns the inheritance of this disease, as it is a common opinion that this condition is genetically transferred. One can simply respond yes, and this is the easiest reply that a doctor can give to concerned patients. However, if the matter is being considered more in depth, another answer might be more indicated. It should be stressed that in the case of inguinal hernia there is not a direct inherited cause for the development of an inguinal protrusion, rather, it is the shape of the pelvis that is being handed down from parents to children. A particular shape of the pelvis forms the main, but not the sole, predisposing factor for the development of an inguinal hernia. Other causes such as professional exposure, comorbidities, smoke, specific sports, or other environmental factors can facilitate the development of a groin hernia in predisposed individuals. By examining the reasons in detail for the pathogenetic involvement of the pelvic shape in determining inguinal protrusions disease, the first consideration to be made is why more than 90% of inguinal hernia patients are male. This undisputable fact could lead us to imagine that there is a significant difference between the two genders concerning the shape of this area and specifically the pelvis shape. To explain this concept, it is essential to have good knowledge of the anatomy of the complex bony district composing the distal half of the human trunk.

G. Amato, *Inguinal Hernia: Pathophysiology and Genesis of the Disease*, https://doi.org/10.1007/978-3-030-95224-2_2

2.2 Anatomy of the Pelvis

The pelvis joins the axial skeleton to the lower limbs. It is composed of a central, posterior pillar constituted by the os sacrum and the coccyx, the paired structures of the ilium that continue on both sides with the hip, the ischium, and pubis bone (Figs. 2.1 and 2.2) [1].

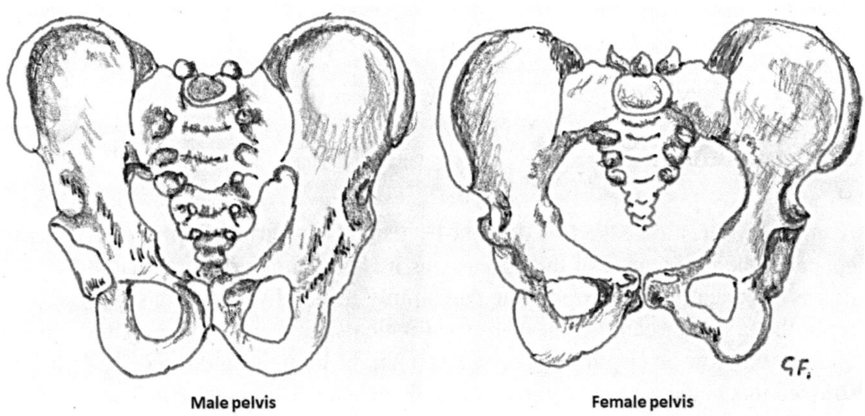

Fig. 2.1 Pelvis shape in males and females: frontal view. The male pelvis has a conic, narrower inlet while the female pelvis is cylindrical with broad empty space © G. Ficile

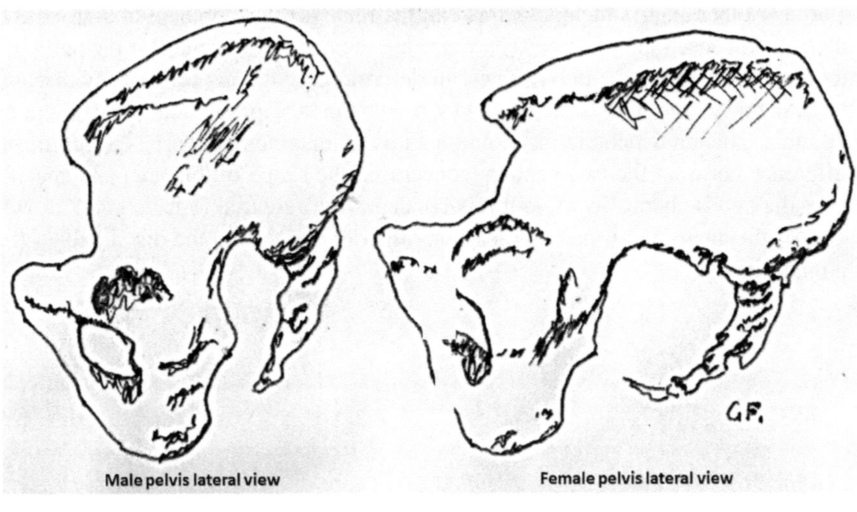

Fig. 2.2 Pelvis shape in males and females: lateral view. Of note, the broad elongated ilium bone of female subjects contrasts with the narrower one of males. Moreover, the sacrococcygeal joint of women is positioned further back than in men © G. Ficile

The sacral bone is a triangular-shaped structure that incorporates the sacral vertebrae S1–S5. It is articulated cranially with the fifth lumbar vertebra and distally to the coccyx, while laterally it is connected to the wing of ilium forming the iliosacral joint.

The coccyx constitutes the most distal part of the vertebral column and is connected to the caudal surface of the os sacrum. It is composed of a variable number of rudimental vertebrae, from 3 to 5. While at first glance, it may resemble an insignificant bony element, the coccyx is the site of insertion of many important myotendineal structures of the lower abdominal area: levator ani, coccygeus, iliococcygeus, and pubococcygeus muscles are inserted in the anterior side. Its posterior surface is connected to the gluteus maximus. Furthermore, the anterior and posterior sacrococcygeal ligaments, the sacrospinous and sacrotuberous ligaments, as well as the lateral sacrococcygeal ligaments, are inserted over the surface of this caudal osseous appendix of the vertebral column [2, 3].

The ilium is a large flat bone that shields the posterior lower abdominal cavity. On its ventral side, close to the iliosacral joint, the posterior iliac spine is located that continues in the cranial, superior side with the iliac crest. This round contoured crest bends and enlarges anteriorly forming the tubercle of the iliac crest, which ends in the anterosuperior iliac spine (ASIS). In its larger portion, the flat body of the ilium descends caudally forming the hip that contains the acetabulum, which articulates with the femur head. Then the hips are joined:

(a) Obliquely in the posterior direction to form the arcuate shape of the ischium.
(b) Anteriorly at the pubic bones that merge in the midline forming the pubic symphysis.

The pubic tubercle, a small promontory that serves as insertion of the inguinal ligament, is located close to the pubic symphysis, which, connected with the ASIS, forms the structure that divides the inguinal and the femoral area [3]. The junction of the pubic bones with the ischium is referred to as the pubic arch and outlines the obturator foramen through which the homonymous muscle as well as the obturator artery, the obturator vein, and the obturator nerve pass.

2.3 Anatomical Differences of the Pelvis Bones between Male and Female

The main anatomical differences between the male and female bony pelvis can be summarized as follows:

Females have a round/oval, and males a conic (heart shaped), pelvic inlet. In particular, the female infra-pelvic space has no obstacle, while on the contrary the

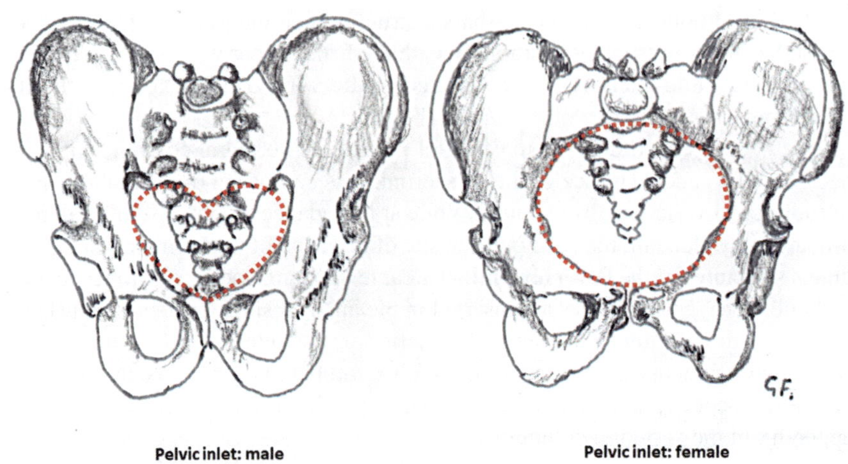

Fig. 2.3 Differences of the pelvic inlet between men and women: in male individuals, the pelvic cavity is narrow, conic, heart shaped. A protuberant sacral promontory further reduces the width of the reservoir. The female pelvis, predisposed for childbearing and passage of the fetus during birth, shows a wide, cylindrical pelvic cavity with no obstacles in its space © G. Ficile

sacral promontory posteriorly obstructs the male pelvis (Fig. 2.3). These significant differences clearly indicate that in females, for facilitating childbearing and fetal passage during birth, no obstacle should be interposed in the bony frame of the lower abdomen [4].

Other minor differences in the pelvic structure between sexes are:

- The iliac spine is higher in males than in females.
- The os sacrum in men is more elongated and narrower compared to women.
- The coccyx in men is fixed and more pronounced in the anterior direction while in women it is mobile and can be dislocated backward.
- The infrapubic arc in men is acute, measuring ca 70° while in women it ranges between 90° and 100°.
- In women, the acetabulum is projected more anteriorly than in men, this anatomical aspect characterizes the typical gait of women.
- The obturator foramen in men shows a round outline but in women it is oval.

Practically, in legal medicine the shape of the pelvis constitutes significant proof for identifying the sex of a cadaver. This means that a more elongated, narrow, and heavier pelvic structure indicates a male pelvis. On the contrary, a wider, lighter pelvis characterizes female individuals. These dissimilarities in width and weight are considered the reason for the different orthostatic attitudes of the human genders since male individuals have a heavier body and therefore need a more robust framework. Furthermore, locomotor behavior between the two sexes is clearly different, and this is quite evident in athletic sports performances [5, 6].

2.4 Significance of Gender-Related Anatomical Difference in the Development of Visceral Protrusions

By taking into account the shape of the pelvis, it is worth noting the physiological events that occur within this anatomical reservoir surrounded by ligaments and multiple layers of muscles. Above all, particular attention should be paid to both static and dynamic phenomena that take place in the abdominal compartment. Steady vector forces originating from the orthostatic pressure exerted by the visceral contents inside the abdominal wall constitute one important feature that characterizes the physiology of this area. Together with orthostatic pressure forces, the digestive function and related production of intestinal gas lead to continuous changes in abdominal pressure. A sudden powerful increase of intraabdominal pressure takes place during coughing or straining. All these phenomena that occur repeatedly can lead to structural changes in the muscular arrangement of the lower abdomen. Actually, by considering the relationship between the forces generated within the abdominal scaffold, it becomes clear that the influence of these forces can have an impact on the structures present therein. It should also be stressed that gender-related differences in the internal pelvic shape may influence the direction of vector forces arising in the abdominal frame. In women, the pelvis is oval and cylindrical without hurdles in its cavity as females are predisposed to childbearing and giving birth (Fig. 2.4).

This means that following gravitational principles, all vector forces generated in the abdominal cavity of females will direct downward toward the pelvic floor. In men, the pelvic cavity is conic with the apex in the caudal portion and partially obstructed by a prominent sacral promontory. This configuration deviates the direction of the orthostatic abdominal vector forces that in males are directed obliquely downward and consequently are bilaterally focused on the groin (Fig. 2.5) [7, 8].

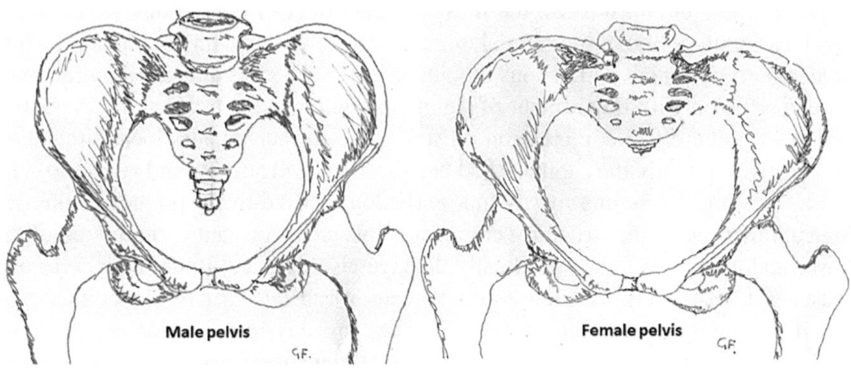

Fig. 2.4 Pelvis shape in males and females: cranio-caudal view: of note, the broad empty space of the female pelvic inlet different from the narrow pelvic infra-bony space of male individuals posteriorly occupied by the sacral promontory © G. Ficile

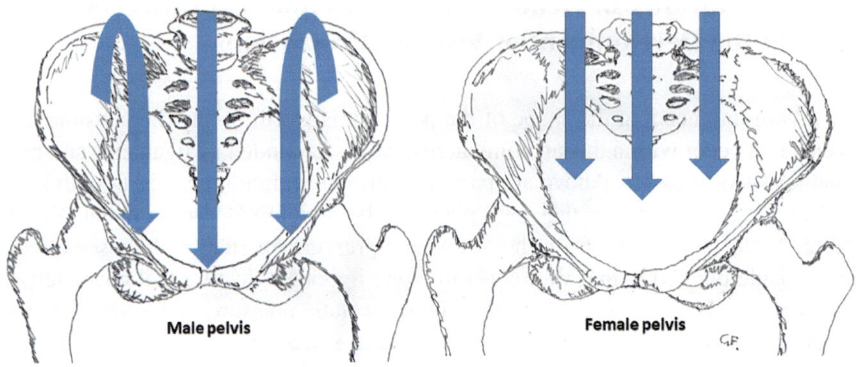

Fig. 2.5 Direction of the orthostatic abdominal pressure forces in men and women. In male individuals, the protuberant sacral promontory obliquely deviates from the caudally directed vector forces. The final target of these forces is the muscle barrier of the inguinal backwall located just above the inguinal ligament. In women, the forces originating in the abdominal cavity cross the practically empty pelvic cavity perpendicularly downward until impact against the muscular structures of the pelvic floor © G. Ficile

2.5 Effects of the Orthostatic Vector Forces upon the Lower Pelvic District

Given the highlighted evidence concerning the physics of the visceral compartment contained inside the abdomen, the results of the effects of these forces upon the physiology of the impacted structures of the lower abdominal wall and the pelvis can be projected. While a steady visceral compression applied upon the solid, hard bony arrangement of the pelvis may have a negligible impact, if these forces are exerted on soft tissues such as the muscular compartment of the lower abdominal cavity it is evident that a series of modifications of the physiology in this area may occur. In these circumstances, the most evident effect of continuous compression involves capillary blood microcirculation, which slows down and is impaired while hindered arterial input and venous output occur [9]. There is also a deterioration of tissue perfusion with impairment of significant biological cell functions. A continued or even increased compression on soft tissue further impairs local circulation and involves not only the capillary bed but also midsized arteries and veins [10, 11]. Aside from the worsening of vascular perfusion that indirectly prejudices physiological functions of the structures composing this area, constant compression of the lower abdominal wall can specifically damage also delicate tissue like nerves and muscles [12–14]. This occurrence initially causes transient structural modifications, but if the compressive impact continues day by day, progressive degeneration including irreversible weakening, leading to complete tissue disbanding, may occur. From a pathogenetic point of view, this degenerative damage, mainly involving the musculature of the pelvic floor as well as the myotendineal arrangement of the lower abdominal wall, is the final effect of a steady orthostatic visceral compression leading to visceral protrusion in predisposed individuals. Specifically, given the broad obstacle-free pelvic inlet that in women directs orthostatic vector forces perpendicularly downward to the pelvic floor, it is easy to understand why a prolapse of visceral organs such as uterus, rectus, and bladder almost exclusively affects female individuals. On the contrary, in male subjects, a prominent sacral promontory that partially obstructs the posterior area of the tightened, conic-shaped pelvic configuration, deviates the orthostatic visceral vector forces obliquely to both sides of the lower anterior abdominal wall. These vector forces specifically directed to the groin, after time, can cause degenerative changes in the musculature of the inguinal barrier, facilitating the development of visceral protrusions.

Considering both the depicted physical phenomena and the different pelvic shapes between the sexes it is easy to understand why inguinal hernia is frequent in men and infrequent in women.

References

1. Eickmeyer SM. Anatomy and physiology of the pelvic floor. Phys Med Rehabil Clin N Am. 2017;28(3):455–60.
2. Foye PM, Patrick M, Buttaci CJ. Coccyx pain. eMedicine 2008.
3. Morris CE. Low Back syndromes: integrated clinical management. McGraw-Hill; 2005. p. 59.
4. Fruchaud H. Anatomic chirurgicale des hernies de l'aine. Paris: Doin; 1956.
5. Vinnicombe SJ, Husband JE. The pelvis. In: Butler P, Mitchell A, Healy JC, editors. Applied radiological anatomy. Cambridge University Press; 2015. p. 279–300.
6. DeSilva JM, Rosenberg KR. Anatomy, development, and function of the human pelvis. Anat Rec (Hoboken). 2017;300(4):628–32.
7. Puntambekar S, Manchanda R. Surgical pelvic anatomy in gynecologic oncology. Int J Gynaecol Obstet. 2018;143(Suppl 2):86–92.
8. Di Gesù G, Greco A, Bellomo S. Fisiopatologia dell'ernia inguinale. Atti 96° Congresso Soc. It. Chir. 1994; 21–37.
9. Park WM, Wang S, Kim YH, Wood KB, Sim JA, Li G. Effect of the intra-abdominal pressure and the center of segmental body mass on the lumbar spine mechanics—a computational parametric study. J Biomech Eng. 2012;134:1.
10. Amato G, Romano G, Salamone G, Agrusa A, Saladino VA, Silvestri F, Bussani R. Damage to the vascular structures in inguinal hernia specimens. Hernia. 2012;16:63–7.
11. Amato G, Calò PG, Rodolico V, Puleio R, Agrusa A, Gulotta L, Gordini L, Romano G. The septum Inguinalis: a clue to hernia genesis? J Investig Surg. 2018;31:1–9.
12. Amato G, Agrusa A, Rodolico V, Caló PG, Puleio R, Romano G. Inguinal hernia: the destiny of the inferior epigastric vessels and the pathogenesis of the disease. Surg Technol Int. 2020;18:36.
13. Amato G, Ober E, Romano G, Salamone G, Agrusa A, Gulotta G, Bussani R. Nerve degeneration in inguinal hernia specimens. Hernia. 2011;15:53–8.
14. Amato G, Agrusa A, Romano G, Salamone G, Gulotta G, Silvestri F, Bussani R. Muscle degeneration in inguinal hernia specimens. Hernia. 2012;16:327–31.

Chapter 3
Physiology of the Inguinal Area

3.1 Introduction

The myotendinous arrangement of the inguinal area constitutes a complex structural and dynamic environment with the function of serving as a barrier for holding the visceral contents within the abdominal cavity. Differently from the rest of the abdominal wall, the inguinal area is characterized by the presence of the inguinal canal that allows the spermatic cord in men and the round ligament in women to cross through, serving as a pathway for the spermatic vessels and ducts. Another peculiar feature of this area is embodied by the different muscular and tendinous compositions. Unlike other portions of the anterolateral abdominal wall, there are only two layers of muscles: the internal oblique and the transverse abdominis. In this context, the external oblique muscle is present as a simple fascial structure that folds in proximate to the inguinal ligament to form the inguinal canal. But the essence of this structural arrangement is represented by the internal inguinal ring that, acting as a true sphincter, plays a crucial role in the physiology and kinetics of the entire groin.

3.2 The Inguinal Sphincter

Also known as the internal or deep inguinal ring, it is formed by interconnected muscular bundles arising from the internal oblique and transverse abdominis muscles; this muscular ring effectively acts as a sphincter-like structure whose action is finalized to impede visceral protrusions into the inguinal canal in the case of raised abdominal pressure. Its sphincter-like behavior was first hypothesized by Jacob Henle who coined the term "Henle'sche Schleife" (Henle's sling) in the mid-nineteenth century [1]. The theory of the inguinal sling was then further confirmed

G. Amato, *Inguinal Hernia: Pathophysiology and Genesis of the Disease*,
https://doi.org/10.1007/978-3-030-95224-2_3

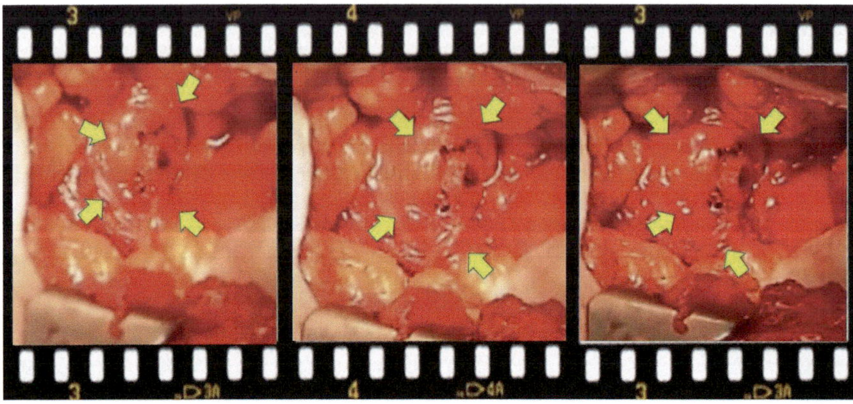

Fig. 3.1 Photographic sequence taken during indirect inguinal hernia repair in local anesthesia. The procedure was carried out with the ProFlor technique. After positioning the 3D scaffold ProFlor within the herniated inguinal sphincter the patient is invited to cough. The images sequentially demonstrate the forceful concentric contraction of the inguinal sphincter (yellow arrows) that squeezes and partially surmounts the structure of the 3D scaffold

one century later by Lytle and commonly accepted in literature [2, 3]. However, the hypothesis of a sling-mimicking contraction of the deep ring was recently visually analyzed, further specified, and detailed by observational studies in vivo carried out during inguinal hernia repair in local anesthesia. This investigational experience evidenced that the contractile function of the internal inguinal ring features not an eccentric, but a concentric muscular contraction identical to that of other sphincter structures, e.g., the anal sphincter [4]. In healthy individuals, in the case of a sudden increase of abdominal pressure, this mode of action allows for restraining of the visceral contents assuring effective protection to the spermatic cord and contained structures. Nevertheless, if for diverse reasons the sphincterial function of this muscular structure is weakened or even impaired, continuous impact of the abdominal viscera against a less competent sphincter can initially lead to transient, incomplete visceral protrusion. If this condition persists and the muscular structure of the inguinal sphincter progressively weakens, the herniation can gradually enlarge thus progressing into the inguinal canal. This is the typical course of an indirect inguinal hernia that progresses into the inguinal canal [5]. In light of this evidence, the terms "internal inguinal ring" and "deep inguinal ring" do not seem to properly depict the true function of this intricate structure: it is more logical to portray the muscular arrangement as an "inguinal sphincter" (Fig. 3.1).

3.3 Integrated Muscular Features of the Groin

Having described the details of the contractile action of the inguinal sphincter, it becomes necessary to highlight the integrated features of the surrounding muscular structures composing the abdominal wall in the inguinal area. In this respect, the rectus abdominis muscle and its sheath lying at the medial margin of the inguinal area play a subordinate but additional protective role. Actually, the contraction of the rectus abdominis muscle during straining or coughing moves latero-caudally in the direction of the inguinal canal. Some scientists hypothesize that the rectus abdominis muscle and its sheath are lateralized following the contraction of the musculature of the lateral abdominal compartment [6]. However, this contractile muscle dislocation is negligible since it only exceptionally reaches the medial half of Hesselbach's triangle, and specifically, the supravesical inguinal fossa [7, 8]. By analyzing the muscular structures composing the inguinal area from the frontal side, it becomes evident that laterally to the rectus abdominis muscle there are three distinct myotendineal layers that, starting from the deep to superficial planes, are oriented in three directions (Fig. 3.2).

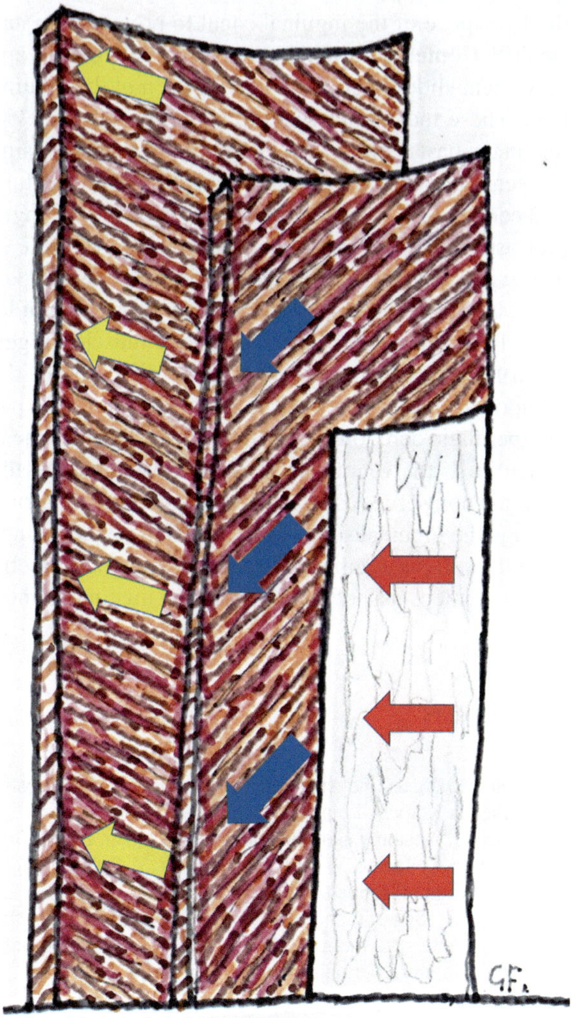

Fig. 3.2 Direction of the vector forces in the inguinal myotendineal structures following muscle contraction (yellow arrows). 1: Transversus abdominis muscle.—2: Internal oblique muscle.—3: External oblique aponeurosis © G. Ficile

The deepest layer is cranially composed of the transversus abdominis muscle and bounded caudally by the iliopubic tract. These two structures are connected together by the transversalis fascia. The internal oblique forms the intermediate compartment. The superficial layer is composed of the aponeurosis of the external oblique muscle. On straining or coughing, the myotendineal structures of the first and the third layer act as a muscular fascia that conveys the opposed motion of the internal oblique muscle [7].

One important contribution in better defining the integrated action of groin muscles in closing off the inguinal sphincter is reported by Skandalakis, who described a significant additional support to the sphincterial motion exerted by the internal oblique and transversus abdominis muscles. Medially of the inguinal sphincter, these two muscles are joined to form the conjoint tendon, which constitutes the medial margin of the inguinal canal. On straining or coughing, thanks to an integrated contraction, this bimuscular compound descends caudally, sharply reducing the free space of the inguinal canal to protect from any attempt of visceral protrusion [9]. Contemporarily, the transversus abdominis aponeurosis with a curtain-like movement slides laterally in the direction of the inguinal ligament and the iliopubic tract. These indications seem to confirm scientific evidence already described earlier, in the past century [10]. Furthermore, opposing simultaneous movements of the myotendineal muscular layers of the groin were postulated in the second half of the past century [11]. The hypothesis of narrowing the inguinal canal to impede visceral protrusion has also been hypothesized [12]. All these coordinated muscular actions triggered by the increase of the abdominal pressure likewise activate the contraction of the cremasteric muscle that retracts, shortening in length and enlarging in thickness. The contraction of the cremasteric muscle triggers another mechanism aimed to further obstruct the inguinal canal: dilatation of the pampiniform plexus. This pseudo-cavernous venous structure, well constituted particularly in the distal half of the spermatic cord, during such an event, activates the arteriovenous capillary shunt system, fills the venous network, and widens more than twice its volume. Such a phenomenon serves as an additional hydrostatic barrier to avoid visceral protrusion through the inguinal sphincter [13]. All these intriguing integrated phenomena demonstrate well the complexity of the physiological mechanisms involved in maintaining the homeostasis of the multifaceted inguinal compound.

References

1. Henle J. Allgemeine Anatomie: Lehre von den Mischungs- und Formbestandteilen des menschlichen Körpers. Leipzig: Voss; 1841.
2. Lytle WJ. Anatomy and function in hernia repair. Proc R Soc Med. 1961;54:967–70.
3. Prescher A, Lierse W. In: Schumpelick V, Nyhus LM, editors. Anatomie der vorderen Leibeswand in Hernien. Thieme Verlag; 2000. p. 16–7.
4. Amato G, Sciacchitano T, Bell SG, Romano G, Cocchiara G, Lo Monte AI, Romano M. Sphincter-like motion following mechanical dilation of the internal inguinal ring during indirect inguinal hernia procedure. Hernia. 2009;13:67–72.

5. Amato G, Marasa L, Sciacchitano T, Bell SG, Romano G, Gioviale MC, Lo Monte AI, Romano M. Histological findings of the internal inguinal ring in patients having indirect inguinal hernia. Hernia. 2009;13:259–62.
6. Peiper C, Junge K, Prescher A, Stumpf M, Schumpelick V. Abdominal musculature and the transversalis fascia: an anatomical viewpoint. Hernia. 2004;8:376–80.
7. Kovachev L, Tonchev P. The groin physiology revisited. International Journal of Clinical Medicine. 2014;5:741–51.
8. Rizk NN. Muscles of the abdomen. In: Williams PL, Warwick R, Dyson M, Bannister LH, editors. Gray's anatomy. 37th ed. New York: C Livingstone; 1989. p. 595–604.
9. Skandalakis JE, Colborn GL, Androulakis JA, Skandalakis LJ, Pemberton LB. Embryologic and anatomic basis of inguinal herniorrhaphy. Surg Clin North Am. 1993;73(4):799–836.
10. Keith A. On the origin and nature of hernia. Br J Surg. 1924;11:455–75.
11. Zimmerman LM. Recurrent inguinal hernia. Surg Clin North Am. 1971;51:1317–24.
12. Donahue PE. Theoretic aspects of hernia. In: Nyhus LM, Condon RE, editors. Hernia. 3rd ed. Philadelphia: J.B. Lipp Co.; 1989. p. 65–73.
13. Hahn-Pedersen J, Lund L, Hønus JH, Bojsen-Møller F. Evaluation of direct and indirect inguinal hernia by computed tomography. Br J Surg. 1994;81(4):569–72.

Chapter 4
Pathological Anatomy and Histology of the Herniated Groin

4.1 Introduction

Over the years, despite the frequency of the disease, very few researchers have dealt with the genesis of inguinal hernia [1, 2]. For much time, there has been no consensus in the scientific community concerning the pathogenetic factors involved in hernia genesis. In the past three decades, an interesting hypothesis considered collagen tissue modifications and related molecular changes as a decisive factor involved in hernia genesis. Altered collagen type I/III ratio was evidenced, but the link between these findings and the development of inguinal protrusions was not proven [3–6]. Therefore, although interesting, this line of thought until now has not proven effective for demonstrating the pathogenetic roots of the disease. In recent years, also the relationship between matrix metalloproteinase (MMPs) and tissue inhibitor metalloproteinase (TIMP) has been hypothesized as having a role in the development of inguinal hernia [7–9]. Nevertheless, a concrete relationship between these biochemical modifications and the development of inguinal protrusions has not been found. It should also be stressed that the theories of collagen type I/III ratio and MMPs/TIMP only consider ultrastructural features of the inguinal substrate, without taking into consideration what effectively happens inside the structural arrangement of the main tissue components of the groin: muscles, vessels, and nerves. This means that these studies have been focused on ascertaining only the ultrastructural changes of the inguinal area without investigating what happens in the structure of the tissue components of the groin where these biochemical phenomena occur. From a rational point of view, it is hard to understand how simply investigating a single biochemical element of a diseased complex structure like the groin can lead to a solid, unconfutable result. In light of these considerations, a series of studies, aimed at outlining type and features of the modifications occurring in the inguinal barrier when a hernia protrusion progresses, has been carried out. Biopsy specimens were

G. Amato, *Inguinal Hernia: Pathophysiology and Genesis of the Disease*,
https://doi.org/10.1007/978-3-030-95224-2_4

gathered with a defined scheme for histological examination finalized to demonstrate eventual existing damage to single tissue elements of the herniated groin, not to the biochemical substrate. The histological study was focused on ascertaining modification of the main tissue elements composing the structure of the inguinal area in detail: muscles, vessels, and nerves [11–16]. The stained specimens were then compared with tissue biopsies excised following the same protocol from the groin of fresh cadavers without inguinal hernia. The results of this investigational experience are noteworthy, above all as this was the first scientific research that successfully determined what really happens within every single element of the inguinal barrier affected by hernia disease. Thanks to these findings, it was possible to ascertain the course of the changes in the myotendineal structure of the groin during the various stages of hernia progressions. In brief, it was finally possible to histologically characterize the type of tissue damage that progressively opens the door to visceral herniation across the lower abdominal wall: a multicomponent degenerative injury with the typical trait of chronic compressive damage.

4.2 The Protocol of Histological Investigation in the Herniated Groin

The above-mentioned studies were carried out by means of biopsy excision in patients who underwent primary inguinal hernia repair and in fresh cadavers with untreated inguinal hernia [10–16]. All types of hernias (direct, indirect, supravesical, combined) were analyzed. To achieve statistically comparable data, tissue samples for histological examination were removed from the structures close to and surrounding the hernia opening following a specific protocol. This involved biopsy removal from tissue corresponding to the same zones in all individuals in the cohort. Independently of hernia type encountered, a vertical line was drawn from the center of the protrusion to the upper border of the defect; from here, two lines diverging at 45° to the right and left were further drawn in a vertical direction above the conjoint tendon. Distances along these lines of 0.5, 1.5, and 2.5 cm away from the border were measured and a full-thickness biopsy of ca 0.5 cm^2 was taken at each of these points along both lines (Fig. 4.1). Even though the described schema did not represent a perfect solution, it was possible to achieve an acceptable mapping of the inguinal area surrounding the protrusion. The same protocol was used for gathering tissue specimens from control cadavers where the midpoint of the conjoint tendon was considered the point of reference for distance assessment of the biopsies. Once the tissue sampling had been carried out, all tissue specimens were fixed in 10% neutral buffered formalin for at least 12 h. After routine tissue processing, the tissue specimens were stained with hematoxylin and eosin (H&E) and PAS for preliminary evaluation. For specific tissue assessment, the following immunohistochemistry

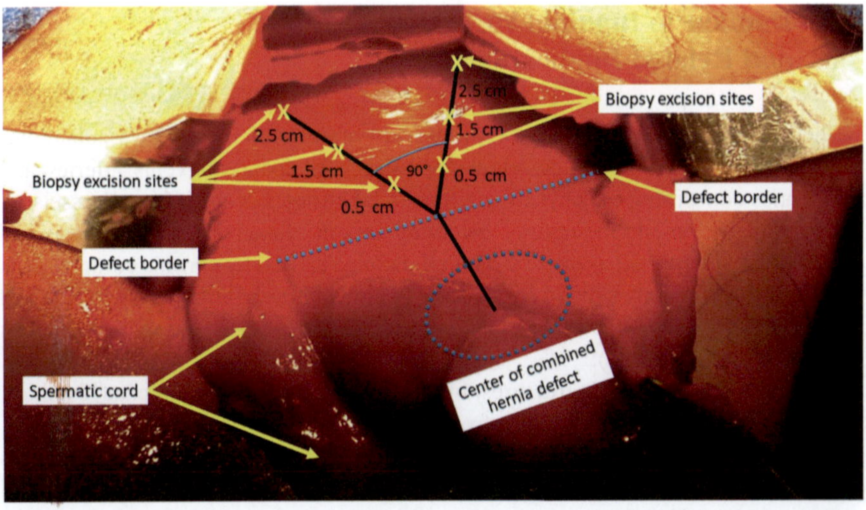

Fig. 4.1 Schematic representation of the biopsy excision sites for histological examination of the inguinal structures involved in hernia protrusion: a line is drawn starting from the center of the protrusion (in this case a large bicomponent combined hernia with direct + indirect components). Two further lines diverging at 45° are drawn in a vertical direction at the junction of this line with the upper border of the defect. Distances along these lines of 0.5, 1.5, and 2.5 cm away from the border were measured. Full-thickness biopsy of ca 0.5 cm^2 was removed along both lines at each of these points

methods were used: Azan Mallory trichrome staining to evidence connective and muscular tissue, CD20, and Factor VIII for vascular elements and NSE for nervous structures.

4.3 Analysis of Histological Findings

The examined specimens revealed a progressive, noteworthy alteration of the structural arrangement in the inguinal area indicating that, starting from the excision point closer to the hernia defect, all encountered tissue elements of the inguinal floor were involved in significant modifications of the normal architecture.

Each specific tissue component of the groin revealed a various degree of damage, which did not always depend on the distance of the excised specimen from the edge of the hernia defect. However, even if to different degrees, a common element characterized these findings: the constant evidence of a chronic inflammatory infiltrate, generally composed of lympho-histiocytes and plasma cells, revealing the presence of a persistent inflammatory process. Apart from basic histological evaluation with H&E, from immunochemistry it was possible to obtain important data concerning the status of the main elements of this area: vessels, muscles, and nerves.

4.4 Damage to Inguinal Vascular Structures and Related Implications

In the examined tissue samples, several types of injuries affecting the vascular components of the groin could be detected: direct structural damage to veins, arteries, and lymphatics concerning the physiologic functional changes of the affected vessels.

Specifically, among the injuries involving venous elements parietal fibrosis and ectasia were interpreted as direct structural damage caused by chronic compression. In addition, the venous network, and more specifically the capillary system, showed clear signs of perivascular edema and congestion due to stasis and reduced venous output (Figs. 4.2 and 4.3).

Concerning the arterial structures, much more evident and significant histological changes can be reported. Aside from a discrete level of parietal fibrosis, a constant hyperplasia of the muscularis tunica leading to thickening of the media was detected among the arteries (Figs. 4.1–4.4). These modifications of the arterial structure were often encountered and, in some case, were so evident as to depict a luminal sub-occlusion or even a manifest occlusion (Figs. 4.5).

These noteworthy alterations of the arterial architecture were documented in a context of obvious sufferance of neighboring tissue, target of the arterial blood perfusion. Muscle fibers and nerves were, in particular, found showing various degrees of structural worsening. In addition, also lymphatic vessels showed manifest alterations, mainly interstitial thickening due to chronic fibrosis, causing irregular endothelial coverage (Fig. 4.6).

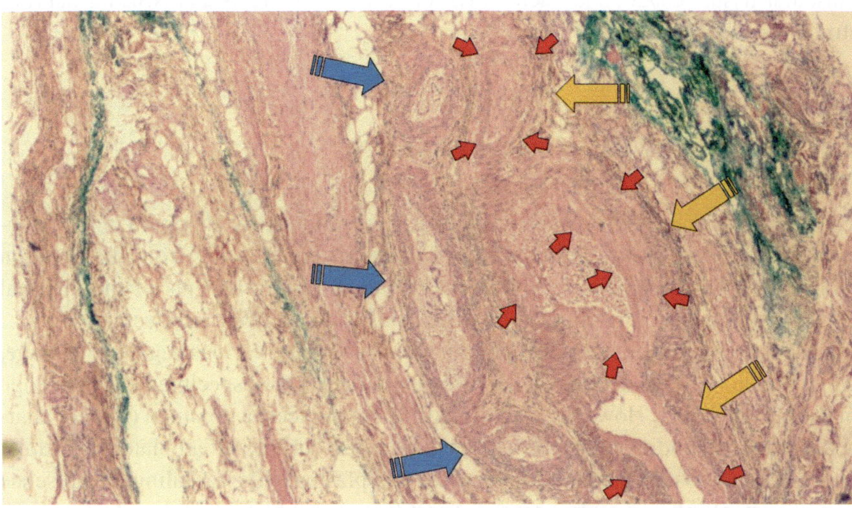

Fig. 4.2 Biopsy specimen excised 0.5 cm from the edge of combined inguinal hernia. Evident parietal fibrosis, ectasia, and stasis of the veins (blue arrows). Tunica media of the arteries (yellow arrows) appears significantly thickened, resulting in a marked reduction of arterial lumen. Findings are consistent with chronic compressive damage. H&E 25X—Reprinted with permission from Amato G.: Springer—Amato G, Romano G, Salamone G, Agrusa A, Saladino VA, Silvestri F, Bussani R. Damage to the vascular structures in inguinal hernia specimens. Hernia 2012;16:63–67

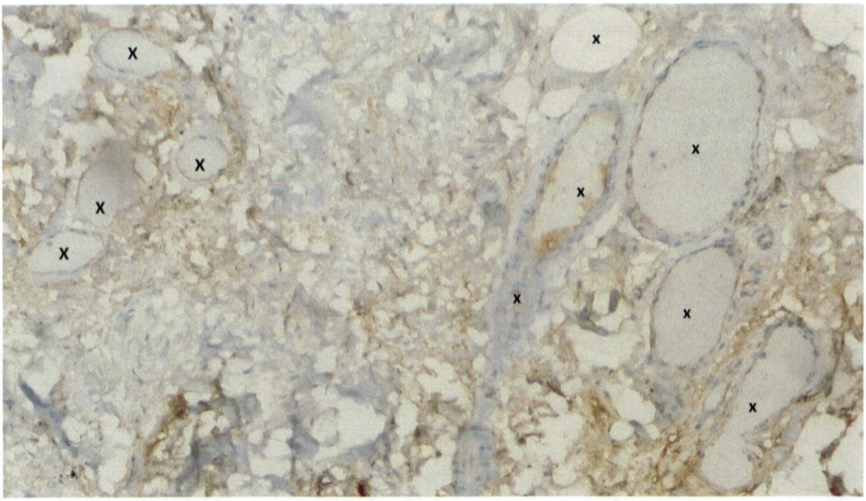

Fig. 4.3 Biopsy excised 1.5 cm from direct inguinal hernia border: convoluted ectatic venous structures (X) as commonly seen in the case of extrinsic compression. The parietal structures of the veins show fibrotic thickening. Factor VIII 100x

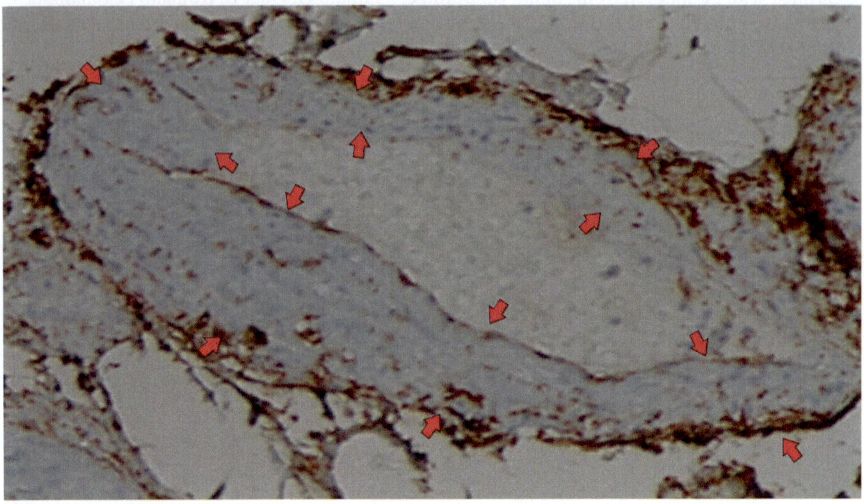

Fig. 4.4 Biopsy excised 1.5 cm from direct hernia edge: midsized arterial structure showing noteworthy thickening of tunica media (red arrows) with consequent reduction of artery lumen. CD31 100×

These findings, with the typical trait of chronic compressive damage, were documented in all herniated patients regardless of hernia type and site of excision; only the degree of damage varied. None of the reported pathological changes to the vascular structures in individuals with hernia were seen in the control specimens excised from cadavers. Analysis of the evidenced changes in the vascular district and specifically venous congestion and arterial stenosis clearly indicates a reduced

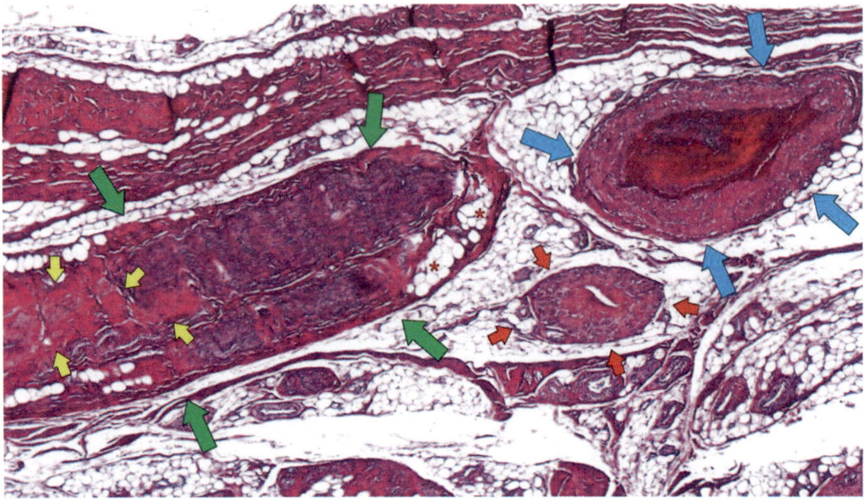

Fig. 4.5 Biopsy excised 2.5 cm from the edge of direct inguinal hernia—Large nervous trunk (green arrow) showing clear degenerative fibrotic dystrophy (yellow arrows) and fatty substitution of the axons (*) in a surround of fatty dystrophy of the muscle fibers. Artery with endoluminal thrombus (blue arrows), arterial sub-occlusion due to media hyperplasia (red arrows)—HE x100—Reprinted with permission from Amato G.: Springer – Amato G, Ober E, Romano G, Salamone G, Agrusa A, Gulotta G, Bussani R. Nerve degeneration in inguinal hernia specimens. Hernia 2011;15:53-58

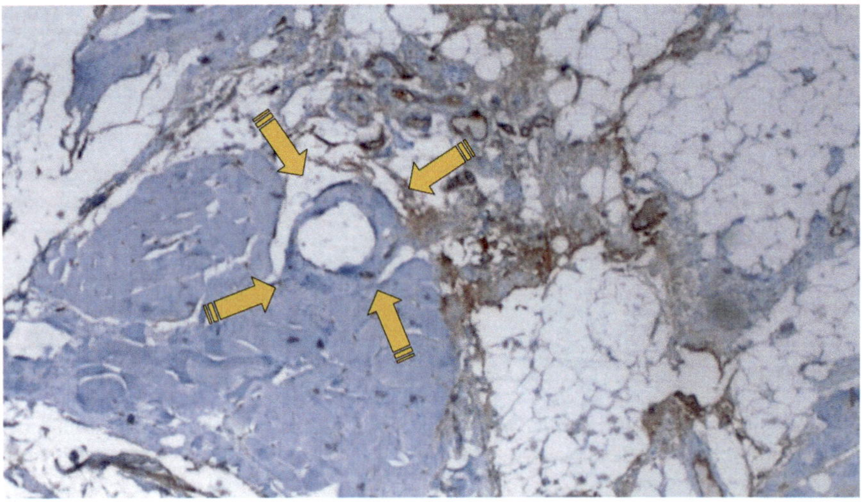

Fig. 4.6 Biopsy specimen excised 1.5 cm from indirect hernia defect: Midsized lymphatic vessel (red arrows) showing ectasia as per upstream compression. The parietal structure of the lymphatic vessel is clearly thickened and partly vacuolized. The endothelial layer is irregular and, in some parts, missing completely. Factor VIII 100×

blood flow to the groin structures. Beyond the modification of the vessel arrangement, a constant finding was a plasma-lymphocytic infiltrate, a typical element of chronic inflammation. This is often connected with persistent compression that affects several anatomical and physiologic mechanisms that normally contribute to homeostasis and maintains the integrity of the inguinal barrier [11].

4.5 Structural Damage Occurring in the Nervous Network of the Inguinal District

Nerve impulse is an essential element of muscle physiology. Impaired or decreased transmission of the nervous impulse seriously affects the contractile action of myocytes leading to weakened motor function. If the deficient functionality of the nervous network progresses over time, also an atrophic involution of the muscle fibers with decreased muscular mass has to be taken into consideration. Histological investigations focused on evidencing structural modifications occurring in nerves of the inguinal area when affected by hernia protrusion have demonstrated a wide spectrum of damage. Tissue specimens removed from this area, which is characterized by the presence of several motor nerves, demonstrated fibrotic degeneration, atrophy, as well as focal fatty dystrophy of the axons (Figs. 4.5 and 4.7).

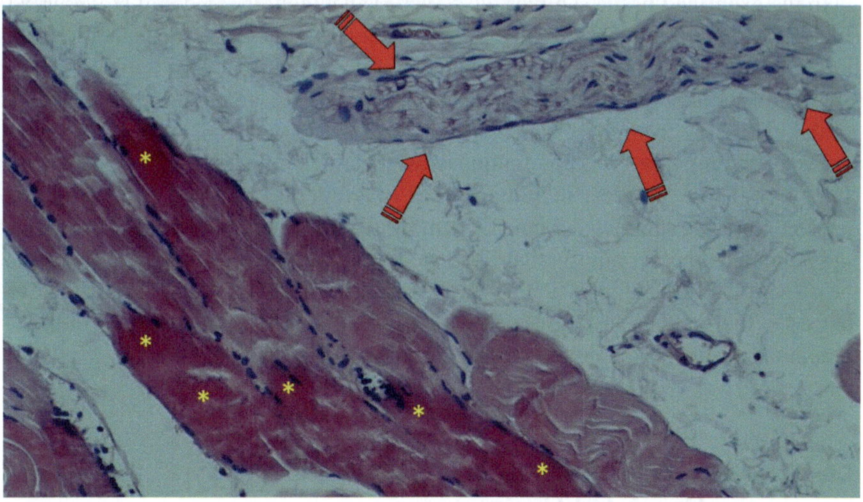

Fig. 4.7 Tissue sample excised at ca 1 cm from the border of direct hernia: muscle bundles showing fibrotic (colored in pale red) and hyaline degeneration (yellow asterisks) surrounded by inflammatory clusters (black spotty elements). Nerve in longitudinal section with manifest edema (red arrows) and atrophy of the axons. PAS 100 Reprinted with permission from Amato G.: Springer – Amato G, Agrusa A, Romano G, Salamone G, Cocorullo G, Mularo S A, Marasa S, Gulotta G. Histological findings in direct inguinal hernia. Hernia 2013;17:757–63

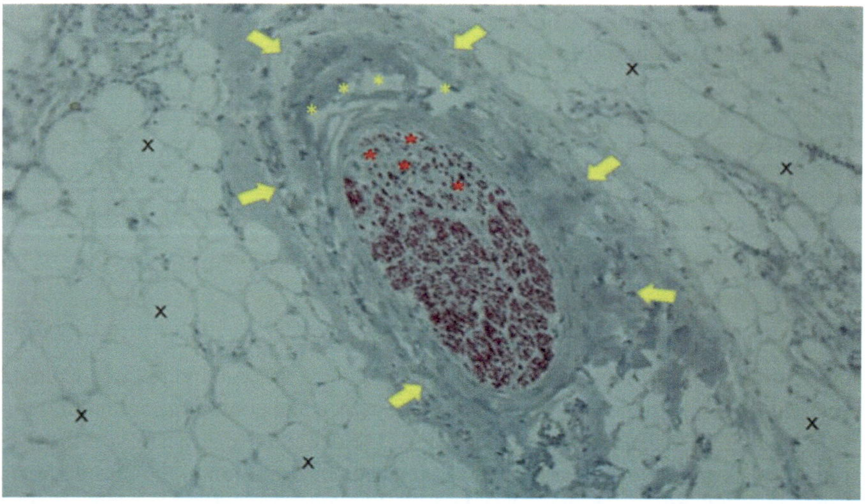

Fig. 4.8 Biopsy specimen excised 0.5 cm from the border of indirect hernia. Fibrotic degeneration of the nerve axons (red asterisks). The myelin sheath (yellow arrows) surrounded by fibro-adipose muscular dystrophy (X) appears evidently thickened and suffering from advanced degenerative injury following chronic compression (yellow asterisks). NSE x200—Reprinted with permission from Amato G.: Springer—Amato G, Ober E, Romano G, Salamone G, Agrusa A, Gulotta G, Bussani R. Nerve degeneration in inguinal hernia specimens. Hernia 2011;15:53-58

In the examined tissue samples, also Wallerian degeneration could be observed. (Fig. 4.8) This kind of lesion, also known as anterograde nerve degeneration, has been reported in literature as a consequence of degeneration of the axon distal to a site of transection and likely derives from the compressive crushing of the nerve trunk [17]. Aside from these specific injuries of the nerve axons, typical of degenerative worsening, a constant finding was the thickening of the myelin sheath (Fig. 4.9). These injuries, including cases of Wallerian degeneration, were also detected in tissue samples 1.5- and 2.5-cm far from the hernia opening. This potentially excludes the hypothesis that the degenerative damage of the nerves could be the effect of direct compression of the hernia contents. The types of damage evidenced in the nervous structures of the groin have already been evaluated in literature and classified as a consequence of chronic compression [18, 19].

4.6 Histological Evidence of Muscular Injuries in the Herniated Groin

Muscles constitute a fundamental component of the abdominal wall. In the highly motile context of the inguinal area, the function of muscular structures assumes a more significant value. A noteworthy improvement in knowledge of the physiology and biodynamics of the muscle function in the inguinal district has been achieved by

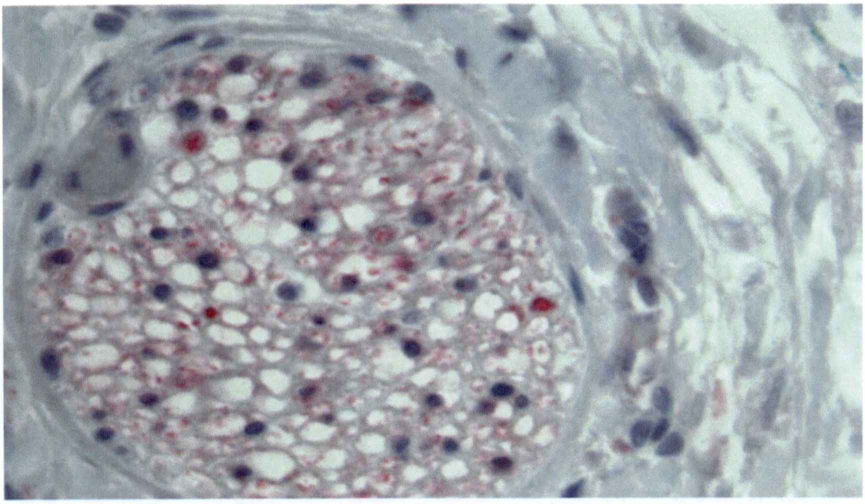

Fig. 4.9 Biopsy specimen excised 1.5 cm from the border of direct inguinal hernia. Wallerian degeneration of a nerve trunk. Almost all nerve axons have disappeared, and Schwann tubes are empty (white spots). The remaining axons show suffering from evident fibrotic degeneration (red spots). Myelin sheath clearly thickened. NSEx630 – Reprinted with permission from Amato G.: Springer – Amato G, Ober E, Romano G, Salamone G, Agrusa A, Gulotta G, Bussani R. Nerve degeneration in inguinal hernia specimens. Hernia 2011;15:53-58

the detailed, also visual, description of the circular squeezing motion of the inguinal sphincter, as seen in Fig. 3.1, which acts as an effective muscular barrier against visceral protrusion [20]. The macroscopic features of the internal ring have already been integrated with histological evidence of biopsy samples removed from this sphincterial arrangement. These tissue specimens clearly revealed why the function of this important muscular structure becomes so impaired as to allow visceral protrusion, thus facilitating the development of indirect inguinal hernia. Muscle atrophy as well as hyaline degeneration, fibrosis, and fatty dysplasia of the myocytes were constantly detected in the tissue specimens removed from the inguinal sphincter at histological examination [21]. Identical injuries of the muscular structure could also be evidenced in every biopsy specimen excised following the biopsy protocol also in other sites and in the case of direct, supravesical or combined hernia. In this context, also vascular and nervous networks which make up the inguinal architecture were found suffering from a specific kind of lesion: degenerative injury with the specific trait of chronic compressive damage. Among inflammatory clusters composed of lympho-histiocytes and plasma cells that were consistently identified close to the damaged muscular structures, muscular atrophy, hyaline, and fibrotic degeneration were frequently documented (Figs. 4.5, 4.7, 4.10, 4.11, 4.12, and 4.13).

Nevertheless, the most frequent degenerative insult identified in the biopsy specimens was fatty dystrophic metaplasia of the muscle fibers (Figs. 4.5, 4.10, 4.11, 4.13). This finding represents the final step of the structural worsening of the myocytes and completes the scale of muscular tissue degeneration. It is frequently

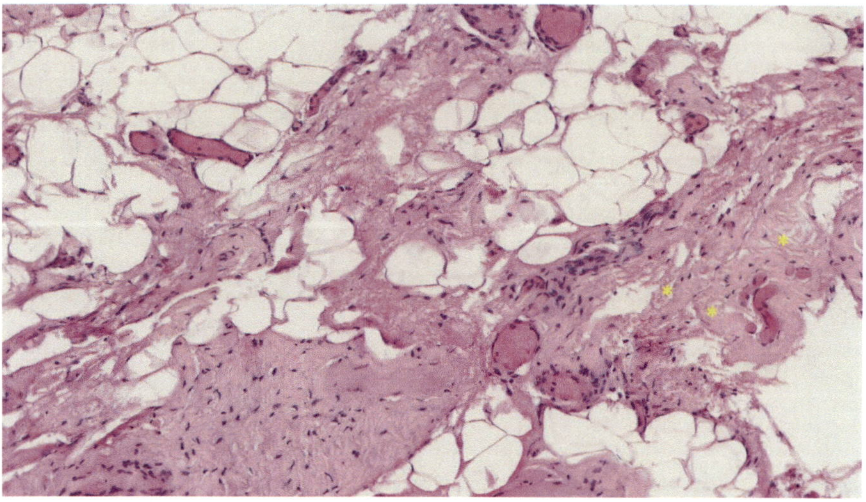

Fig. 4.10 Biopsy specimen excised 2.5 cm from indirect hernia defect: Evidence of severe muscle damage with atrophy, hyaline degeneration, and fibrosis of the muscle bundles (colored in pale red). In this context, several areas of fatty dystrophy of the myocytes (white circular elements), venous ectasia (red spots), and tissue edema (yellow asterisks) emerge. Noteworthy inflammatory infiltrate composed of lymphocytes and plasma cells (black spotty elements) is also visible. EE 100×

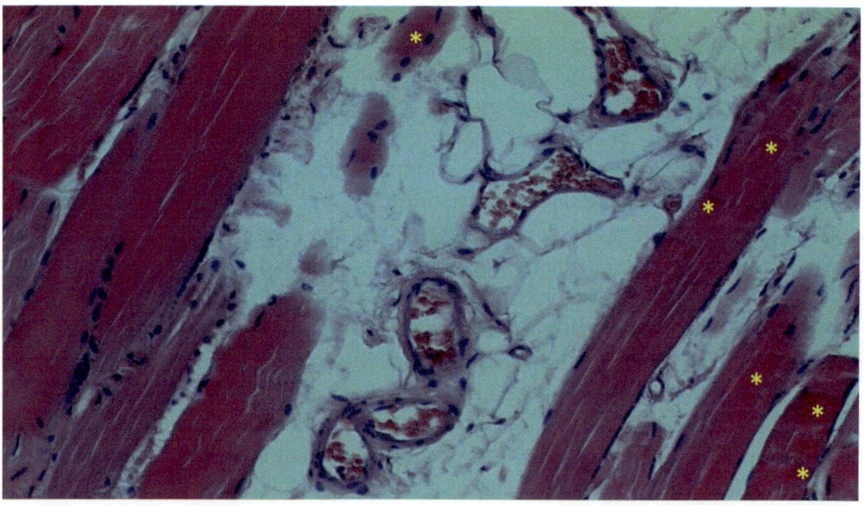

Fig. 4.11 Tissue sample excised at ca 1.5 cm from hernia border: fibrotic (colored in pale red) and hyaline degeneration (yellow asterisk) of the muscle fibers. Fatty muscle dystrophy (white spots). Evident inflammatory infiltration (black spotty elements). Venous ectasia and congestion (red arrows). PAS 200x Reprinted with permission from Amato G.: Springer – Amato G, Agrusa A, Romano G, Salamone G, Cocorullo G, Mularo S A, Marasa S, Gulotta G. Histological findings in direct inguinal hernia. Hernia 2013;17:757–63

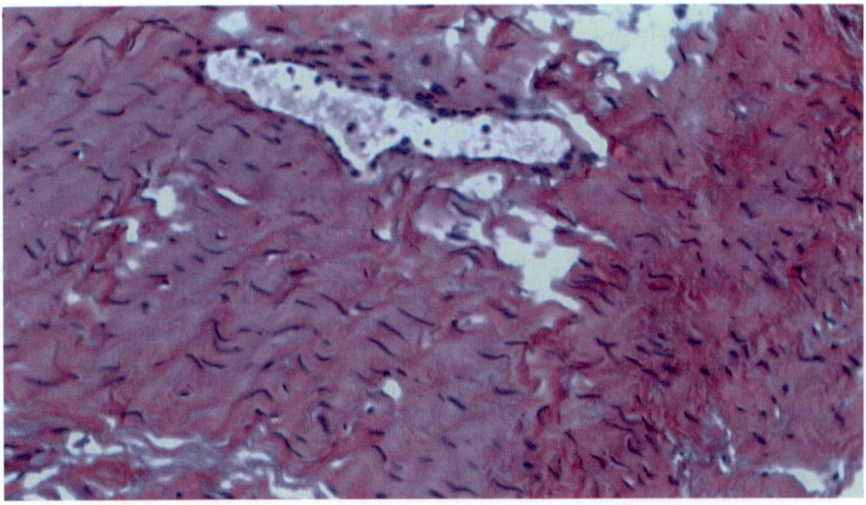

Fig. 4.12 Tissue biopsy excised from the internal ring in a patient affected by indirect inguinal hernia: the microphotograph shows diffuse initial, albeit progressive damage of the myocytes. In the upper quadrant, a midsized vein is evidently enlarged, congested, and surrounded by lymphoplasma cellular infiltrate. HEx200 Reprinted with permission from Amato G.: Springer – Amato G, Marasa L, Sciacchitano T, Bell SG, Romano G, Gioviale MC, Lo Monte AI, Romano M. Histological findings of the internal inguinal ring in patients having indirect inguinal hernia. Hernia 2009;13:259-62

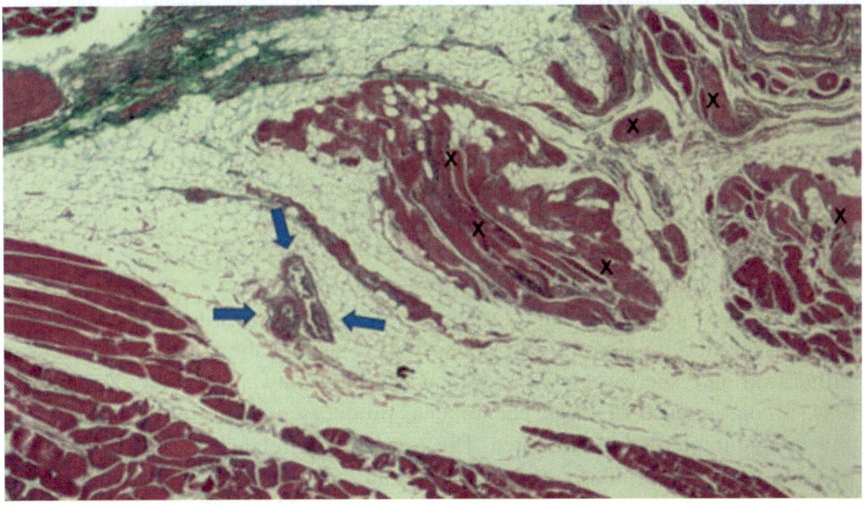

Fig. 4.13 Biopsy specimen excised 2.5 cm from direct hernia border. Massive fatty metaplasia of the muscle bundles (white spotty elements), surrounded by fibrosis of muscle fibers. In the center of the microphotograph a group of small veins appears evidently enlarged and congested (blue arrows). HE x100 Reprinted with permission from Amato G. – Springer - Amato G, Agrusa A, Romano G, Salamone G, Gulotta G, Silvestri F, Bussani R. Muscle degeneration in inguinal hernia specimens. Hernia 2012;16:327-31

described with the same progression in cardiac muscle tissue and originates from tissue ischemia. The pathway of the phenomena sequence occurring in muscle cells, from hypoxia to fatty dystrophy, has already been biochemically confirmed and well established [22, 23]. Furthermore, fatty dystrophy is a well-known aspect of muscle degeneration following chronic ischemia and is frequently reported in heart tissue samples as a consequence of myocardial infarction [24]. Although at first glance these degenerative changes of the myocytes appear identical, as the anatomic substrate is completely different also the pathogenetic source of these injuries varies significantly. Actually, in the cardiac district tissue ischemia is caused by stenosis or obstruction of the coronary arteries, while the etiology of the reported muscle damage in the inguinal area is totally different and can only be justified as an effect of a steady, long-lasting compressive force impacting against the muscular structure. In literature, similar alterations of the muscular structure caused by steady compression have already been confirmed [25].

4.7 Effects of the Histologically Evidenced Damage on the Physiology of Inguinal Structures

The wide range of injuries histologically documented in the diverse tissue structures composing the inguinal barrier exerts significant interconnected worsening effects upon the biodynamics of this district. As described, chronic compressive damage represents the common trait of these lesions. The compression applied to the vascular structures causes direct and indirect damage. The direct impact of compressive forces upon the groin is quite extended, and usually manifests with reduced blood flow affecting direction of the blood flow, both inlet and outlet. Venous ectasia, tissue congestion, and edema, always surrounded by chronic inflammatory clusters, represent a constant finding in the presence of chronic compression [16, 24]. The steady compressive effect upon the arterial layers causes a concentric hyperplasia of the muscular arrangement of the tunica media. Thickening of the media in the arteries leads to sub-occlusion and in some cases to complete occlusion of the arterial lumen. This is also a consequence of persistent compression on the arterial structures. Furthermore, also chronic inflammation is well-known to be a contributing factor in the development of obstructing hyperplasia of the artery which leads to withdrawal and sclerosis of the arteriolar capillary network [26]. Reduced blood flow, a consequence of these phenomena, produces noteworthy anatomical and physiologic impairment in this area. The compression-related reduced arterial inlet causes a lessening of the oxygen supply leading to chronic ischemia, which has a significant metabolic impact. In the long-term, reduced blood flow impairs the metabolic processes leading to morphological changes and stress-induced cellular injury that ultimately weakens the structural defense mechanisms in the tissue elements of the inguinal area. These three factors—inflammation, venous congestion, and arterial obstruction—logically represent an effective source of structural weakening of the abdominal wall in the inguinal area involved in the hernia protrusion. In addition, the lesions of the nerves found in tissue specimens of herniated patients assume a particular role. The structural and functional damage of the nerves resulting from thickening of the myelin sheath, fibrosis, and progressive degeneration of the axons evidently have a negative impact on the end target of the nervous impulse in this area: the muscle barrier of the groin. Diminished or even a complete blockade of the nerve impulse would have a negative effect on the muscle contraction of the highly mobile context of the groin, especially if the protective muscular mechanisms of the inguinal sphincter are being considered. Muscle atrophy following a progressive worsening of the motor impulse to muscle fibers, loss of contractile power, and reduced muscle mass thickness constitute an additional, indirect damage other than direct compression. In literature, these changes in the nervous arrangement are described as a specific consequence of chronic compressive damage [10, 17, 19]. The evidence of vascular and nervous modifications in the inguinal district constitutes a specific adaptation in the framework of the multifactorial disease of inguinal hernia. However, the most important finding of the reported injuries that plays a crucial role in the development of inguinal hernia is the fatty dystrophy of the inguinal backwall. This phenomenon is the ultimate effect of the persistent compression exerted upon the muscular barrier and leads to extended fatty metaplasia of the muscles. In brief, the muscle becomes a fatty stripe clearly unable to contract and unfit to oppose abdominal pressure. At this stage, a simple episode of coughing or straining is sufficient to breach the disbanded muscular curtain allowing the forceful penetration of an abdominal viscus through the inguinal canal.

4.8 Chronic Compression on the Inguinal Barrier Leading to Tissue Degeneration. Which Source?

Histology of the herniated groin, mentioned above, definitely clarifies the condition of all elements composing the herniated inguinal barrier. The cited recent studies have given an enormous impulse in determining the steps of the development of inguinal protrusions and, above all, their true source. In the previous paragraphs of this chapter, the narrative of histological findings was always focused on highlighting the effective damage documented regardless of the source. This is actually the role of the pathologist: describing the microscopic features of the examined tissue specimen in detail. The role of a clinician, who aims to unveil the etiology of a disease in a complex anatomic environment, is different. In the case of inguinal hernia, a profound knowledge of pathological anatomy and histology is not sufficient to center the target, rather a multidisciplinary skill is required. Broad-based experience in the specific gross anatomy, physics, physiology, histology, and surgical anatomy of the inguinal area is essential to achieve the goal of identifying the genesis of this intriguing disease. Based on these principles, the reported histological findings undoubtedly helped in determining the pathogenetic roots of inguinal hernia. The most important finding that concretely addressed the search for the pathogenesis was the identification of a constant element that characterized the sufferance of all inguinal components: the diffused and persistently present signs of chronic compression. At this stage, the question was: how many sources of chronic compression are present in the lower abdominal area? There were not so many choices in answering: only steady visceral impact upon the groin can lead to chronic compression!

Moreover, the statements made in Chap. 2 concerning the difference in the pelvis shape between sexes, as well as the types and frequency of visceral protrusion disease in men and women, further strengthened the idea of orthostatic tissue degeneration being the culprit of visceral herniation/prolapse occurring in both genders.

In light of this evidence, it can be postulated that the highlighted degenerative tissue damage leading to inguinal hernia originates from chronic orthostatic visceral impact.

References

1. Stoppa R. Como se forma una hernia inguinal? Actualizacion en chirugia del aparato digestivo. Fundacion MMA. 1984–2004;8:469–73.
2. Read RC. Recent advances in the repair of groin herniation. Curr Probl Surg. 2003;40(1):13–79. 12
3. Friedman DW, Boyd CD, Norton P, Greco RS, Boyarsky AH, Mackenzie JW, Deak SB. Increases in type III collagen gene expression and protein synthesis in patients with inguinal hernias. Ann Surg. 1993;218(6):754–60.
4. Pans A. Biochemical study of collagen in adult groin hernias. J Surg Res. 2002;95(2):107–13.
5. Klinge U, Binnebösel M, Mertens PR. Are collagens the culprits in the development of incisional and inguinal hernia disease? Hernia. 2006;10(6):472–7. 13
6. Klinge U, Binnebösel M, Rosch R, Mertens P. Hernia recurrence as a problem of biology and collagen. J Minim Access Surg. 2006;2(3):151–4.
7. Jain V, Srivastava R, Jha S, Misra S, Rawat NS, Amlab DV. Study of matrix metalloproteinase-2 in inguinal hernia. J Clin Med Res. 2009;1(5):285–9.
8. Antoniou GA, Tentes IK, Antoniou SA, Simopoulos C, Lazarides MK. Matrix metalloproteinase imbalance in inguinal hernia formation. J Investig Surg. 2011;24(4):145–50.18
9. Isik A, Gursul C, Peker K, Aydın M, Fırat D, Yılmaz I. Metalloproteinases and their inhibitors in patients with inguinal hernia. World J Surg. 2017;41(5):1259–66.
10. Amato G, Ober E, Romano G, Salamone G, Agrusa A, Gulotta G, Bussani R. Nerve degeneration in inguinal hernia specimens. Hernia. 2011;15:53–8.
11. Amato G, Romano G, Salamone G, Agrusa A, Saladino VA, Silvestri F, Bussani R. Damage to the vascular structures in inguinal hernia specimens. Hernia. 2012;16:63–7.
12. Amato G, Agrusa A, Romano G, Salamone G, Gulotta G, Silvestri F, Bussani R. Muscle degeneration in inguinal hernia specimens. Hernia. 2012;16:327–31.
13. Amato G, Agrusa A, Romano G, Salamone G, Cocorullo G, Mularo SA, Marasa S, Gulotta G. Histological findings in direct inguinal hernia. Hernia. 2013;17:757–63.
14. Amato G, Calò PG, Rodolico V, Puleio R, Agrusa A, Gulotta L, Gordini L, Romano G. The septum Inguinalis: a clue to hernia genesis? J Investig Surg. 2018;31:1–9.
15. Amato G, Agrusa A, Rodolico V, Caló PG, Puleio R, Romano G. Inguinal hernia: the Destiny of the inferior epigastric vessels and the pathogenesis of the disease. Surg Technol Int. 2020;18:36.

16. Tozzi P. The physiology of blood flow and artery wall. In: Tozzi P, editor. Sutureless anastromoses: secrets for success. Darmstadt: Springer; 2007. p. 12–24.
17. Penkert G. Nerve compression syndrome-1. Chirurg. 1998;69:1114–22.
18. Kincaid JC. Stewart JD focal peripheral neuropathies. J Clin Neuromuscul Dis. 1999;1(2):113.
19. Kanchiku T, Taguchi T, Kaneko K, Yonemura H, Kawai S, Gondo T. A new rabbit model for the study on cervical compressive myelopathy. J Orthop Res. 2001;19(4):605–13.
20. Amato G, Sciacchitano T, Bell SG, Romano G, Cocchiara G, Lo Monte AI, Romano M. Sphincter-like motion following mechanical dilation of the internal inguinal ring during indirect inguinal hernia procedure. Hernia. 2009;13:67–72.
21. Amato G, Marasa L, Sciacchitano T, Bell SG, Romano G, Gioviale MC, Lo Monte AI, Romano M. Histological findings of the internal inguinal ring in patients having indirect inguinal hernia. Hernia. 2009;13:259–62.
22. Silvestri F, Bussani R. Hypoxic right ventricular cardiomyopathy. A morphological and pathogenetic study on the myocardial atrophy and fatty infiltration. Pathologica. 1990;82:593–616.
23. Basso C, Thiene G, Corrado D, Angelini A, Nava A, Valente M. Arrhythmogenic right ventricular cardiomyopathy. Dysplasia, dystrophy, or myocarditis? Circulation. 1996;94(5):983–91.
24. Bai YH, Takemitsu M, Atsuta Y. Takemitsu Y pathology study of rabbit calf muscles after repeated compression. J Orthop Sci. 1998;3(4):209–15.
25. Boyd GW. The patho-physiology of chronic arterial hypertension: a hypothesis. Clin Exp Pharmacol Physiol. 1980;7(5):541–4.
26. Schoen FJ, Blood vessels. In: Kumar V, Abbas AK, Fausto N, editors. Robbins and Cotran pathologic basis of disease. 7th ed. Philadelphia: Elsevier; 2005. p. 513–5.

Chapter 5
The Septum Inguinalis: Its Role in the Pathogenesis of Inguinal Hernia

5.1 Introduction

Significant histological findings from the herniated groin in recent studies provide a clear clue in establishing steady orthostatic visceral impact upon the myotendineal structure of the inguinal backwall as the source of inguinal hernia disease. The depicted tissue damage has also been documented in biopsy specimens taken some distance from the hernia border. This implies that structural worsening of the inguinal architecture is not caused by compression exerted by the expansion of hernia content, as the protrusion is located at centimeters of distance from the biopsy sites. Nevertheless, additional scientific evidence is needed to indisputably confirm orthostatic visceral impact as the cause of tissue degeneration following chronic compressive damage. A solid opportunity to exclude the compressive effects of the protrusion expansion as a cause of degenerative damage in the groin came from the evidence of a new, previously unknown anatomical structure situated in the inguinal backwall: the septum inguinalis [1]. This anatomical arrangement is visible in a particular type of multiple ipsilateral hernia, the so-called pantaloon hernia, composed of the concomitance of two protrusions in the inguinal area: one direct plus one indirect hernia separated by a strip of tissue, the septum inguinalis. Multiple ipsilateral hernias are relatively frequent, accounting for 10–15% of all hernias [2–6]. In literature, a specific type of hernia, the pantaloon hernia, has been portrayed as the intermediate stage of the evolution of inguinal protrusion disease. It represents the effect of degenerative harm caused by visceral impact concomitantly affecting both the lateral and the medial inguinal fossae. In short, pantaloon hernias merely represent one of various steps in the progression of degenerative insults affecting the inguinal barrier and are preludes to the confluence of these two types of hernias. In effect, the dissolution of the dividing diaphragm leads to a single, unified protrusion: the combined inguinal hernia [7].

G. Amato, *Inguinal Hernia: Pathophysiology and Genesis of the Disease*, https://doi.org/10.1007/978-3-030-95224-2_5

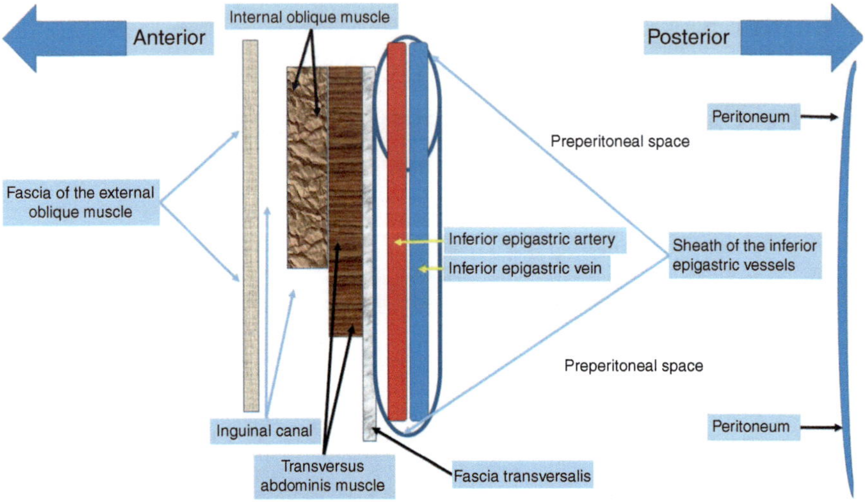

Fig. 5.1 Schematic representation of structures making up the septum inguinalis and neighboring anatomical elements (sagittal view)

5.2 Components of the Septum Inguinalis

The septum inguinalis separates the two protrusions of a pantaloon hernia in a cranio-caudal direction. It is composed of distinct layers of different anatomical structures (Fig. 5.1).

This divisor septum is usually shaped like a trunked cone of muscle bundles with the apex directed downward (Fig. 5.2). The anterior surface is entirely made up of interconnected fibers of the internal oblique muscle and the transversus abdominis (Fig. 5.3). Then, from the anterior to the posterior perspective, the transversalis fascia forms the mid-layer of the diaphragm. The sheath of the inferior epigastric vessels, which enwraps the homonymous vascular elements that perpendicularly cross the inguinal backwall, is found attached to the posterior surface of the transversalis fascia, in the preperitoneal space (Fig. 5.4). In surgical anatomy, these mid-sized vessels originating from the femoral artery and vein form the boundary between the lateral and medial inguinal fossa and historically constitute the lateral margin of Hesselbach's triangle [8].

5.3 Gross Anatomical Modifications of Septum Inguinalis in the Herniated Groin

The multi-structured arrangement of the septum inguinalis is subjected to progressive modification of its components over time in the presence of the specific condition of pantaloon hernia. These phenomena, both macro- and microscopically, show

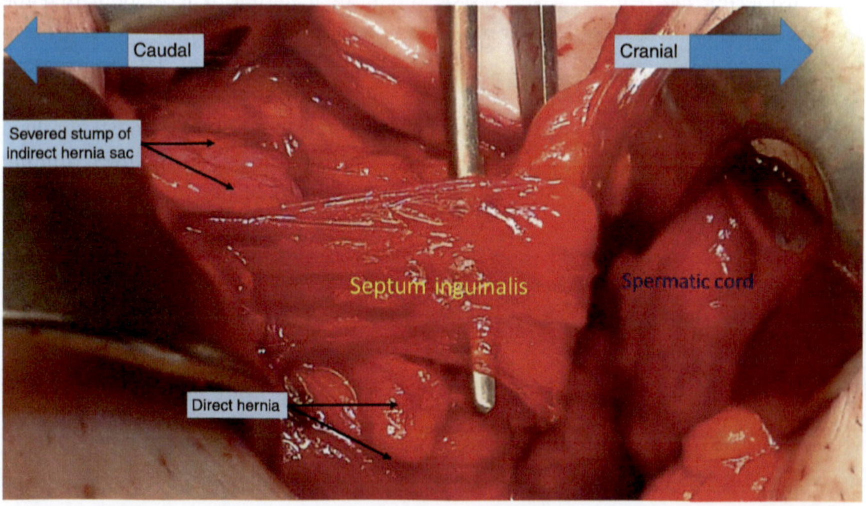

Fig. 5.2 Photo taken during an open anterior inguinal hernia repair procedure. The image shows a septum inguinalis interposed between a direct and an indirect hernia. The trunked conic shape of the longitudinally oriented muscle bundles that form the anterior portion of the septum is evident

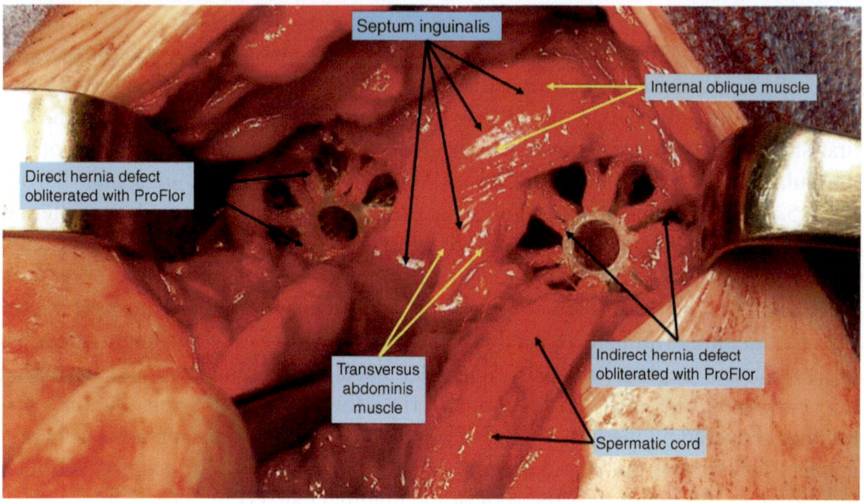

Fig. 5.3 Photo taken during an open anterior inguinal hernia repair procedure in a case of double ipsilateral inguinal hernia composed of a direct and an indirect protrusion. Both hernias have already been obliterated with two 25 mm ProFlor dynamic hernia scaffolds that occupy both defects. The image highlights a robust septum inguinalis that separates the defects. This septal arrangement is clearly made up of fibers of the internal oblique muscle in the foreground and of the transversus abdominis muscle in the background

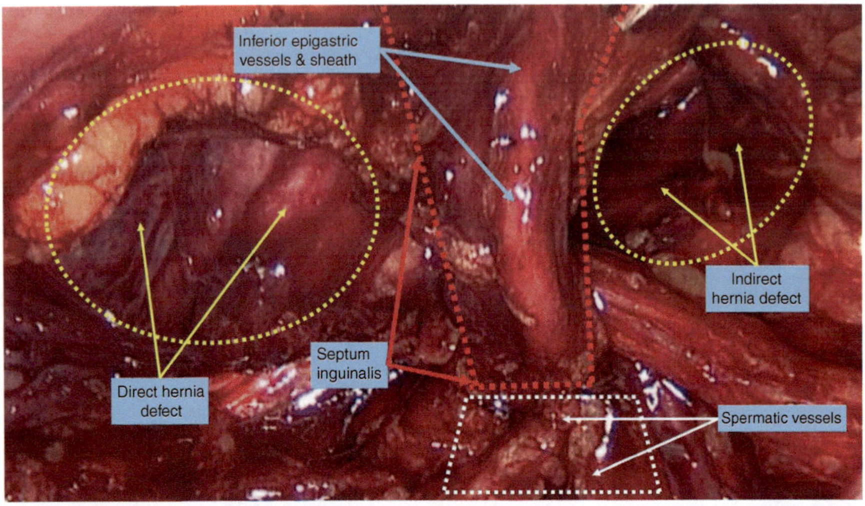

Fig. 5.4 Photo taken during laparoscopic inguinal hernia repair with TAPP technique. The image shows the preperitoneal surface of the posterior abdominal wall in the inguinal area. It documents the presence of a large direct hernia defect that is separated from an indirect hernia defect by the septum inguinalis, indicated by the intermittent red lines. Note prominence of the inferior epigastric vessels and sheath that characterize the posterior, preperitoneal perspective of the septum

the typical damage that derives from a steady compressive force applied upon this area, which is constrained between the visceral content of the abdominal cavity and the robust fascia of the external oblique that anteriorly covers the inguinal area. The first step in the structural modification of the septum inguinalis is atrophy of the muscular layer. From an initial condition of being a robust muscular barrier (Fig. 5.3), the bilayered muscular structure composed of fibers of the internal oblique and the transversus abdominis starts to reduce in thickness, gradually becoming a thin muscular substrate that still covers the epigastric vessels (Fig. 5.5). Over time, the effects of the compressive damage caused by the orthostatic vector forces originating from the visceral compartment continue to increasingly affect the thinner divisor septum until the muscular substrate completely vanishes. This degeneration of the muscular layer anteriorizes the epigastric vessels that only initially are covered by the transversalis fascia. Then, also the transversalis fascia disappears leaving the epigastric vessels fully exposed, facing the external oblique fascia that in this area forms the roof of the inguinal canal (Fig. 5.6).

A progressive structural worsening of the inferior epigastric vessels represents the last step of the depicted degenerative progression stressing the septum inguinalis. Under the effect of steady compression, these vascular elements react with a thickening of the vascular wall. Persistence of the compressive insult reduces both vessels into a small, stiff strip of tissue (Fig. 5.7). After this, steadily subjected to the compressive impact of the abdominal visceral contents, the remains of the septum

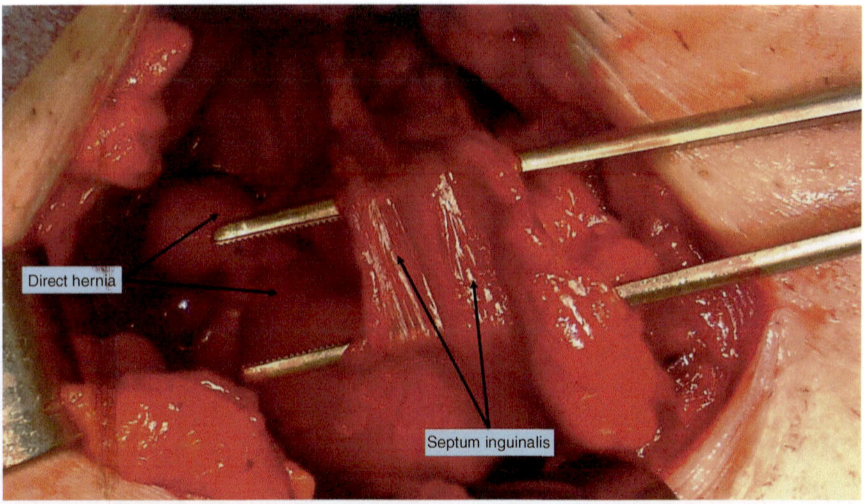

Fig. 5.5 Open anterior inguinal hernia repair procedure in a case of double ipsilateral inguinal hernia composed of a direct and an indirect protrusion (not visible in this image). The septum inguinalis is reduced in width and in thickness, being made up of a thin muscular layer on the anterior side

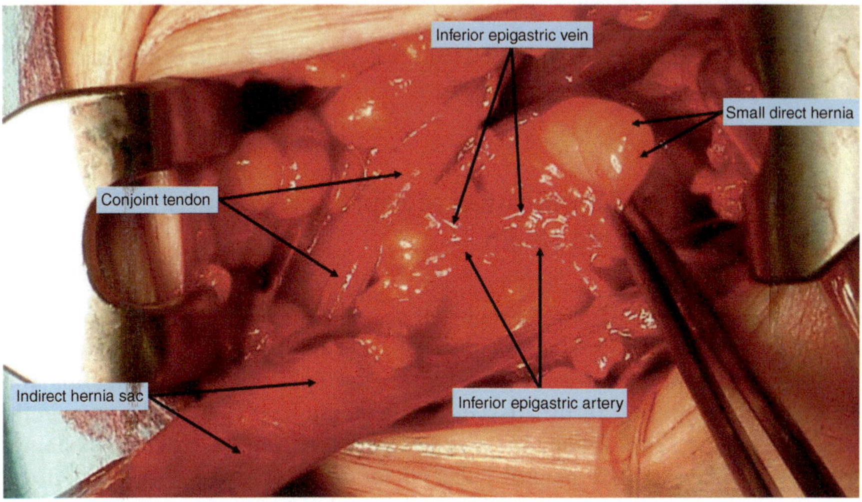

Fig. 5.6 Open anterior inguinal hernia repair procedure in a case of double ipsilateral inguinal hernia composed of a small direct hernia and a large indirect protrusion. The image shows the complete absence of the muscular layer of the septum inguinalis which has fully disintegrated leaving the inferior epigastric vein and artery anteriorized and exposed

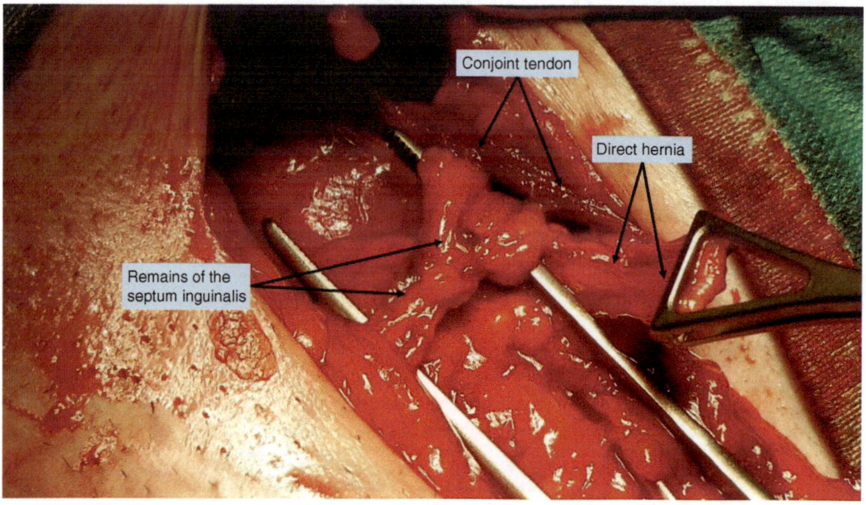

Fig. 5.7 Open anterior inguinal hernia repair procedure for double ipsilateral inguinal hernia made up of two distinct hernias, one direct and one indirect (not visible in this image). The protrusions are separated by thin remains of the septum inguinalis barely containing the inferior epigastric vessels. The image depicts the last stage of the degenerative damage involving the septum inguinalis prior to complete disbanding when the two protrusions are unified in one: the combined inguinal hernia

inguinalis completely disintegrate and vanish, giving birth to a new, unified inguinal protrusion: the combined inguinal hernia.

5.4 Histological Modification of Septum Inguinalis in the Herniated Groin

The degree of macroscopic alteration of the septum inguinalis encountered in several patients suffering from pantaloon hernias urged additional investigation of the microscopic substrate of the septum inguinalis. This investigation was finalized to ascertain if further tissue damage could be histologically seen in the structure of the septa inguinalia. Excised septa were histologically examined after being fixed in 10% neutral buffered formalin, dehydrated in ethanol and paraffin-embedded according to the routine technique; 4–5 μm thick sections were cut and stained with hematoxylin and eosin (HE) for basic histological examination. Immunostaining was carried out with Azan Mallory, and Masson's trichrome was used to highlight collagen and muscular tissue. Further sections were exposed to anti-von Willebrand Factor (Factor VIII) antibody and CD31 immunostaining to highlight vascular structures, while NSE was used for the nervous structures [1, 9].

Histopathological examination of the H&E stained specimens showed manifest degenerative damage of the muscle bundles, including hyaline degeneration, fibrosis, and fatty dystrophy. These pathological findings of the connective tissue could also be seen from immunochemistry (Fig. 5.8).

Concerning the vessels of this district, and in particular the inferior epigastric vessels, hypertrophy of the tunica media of the epigastric artery was constantly found. In some case, the entire arterial wall was found in a stage of advanced degenerative damage with signs of incipient colliquation (Fig. 5.9).

Additional deterioration of the arterial structure in the form of stenotic restriction of the lumen could be segmentally detected in many samples (Fig. 5.10).

Further pathological findings were found concerning the inferior epigastric veins, which demonstrated ectasia and congestion. Some specimens also showed the epigastric vein in a stage of advanced degeneration in a context of inflammatory infiltrate composed of lympho-plasmacellular elements (Fig. 5.9). These signs are consistent with severe circulatory damage. Congestive vasculopathy and medial hypertrophy with arterialization deriving from impairment of blood outflow further emphasized worsening of the vascular support. Concerning the nervous structures, fibrotic degeneration of the nerve axons and thickened myelin sheath was a constant finding, and, in some cases, Wallerian degeneration could be noticed (Fig. 5.11). Overall, the histological findings indicate that all the recognized tissue injuries were consistent with chronic compressive damage.

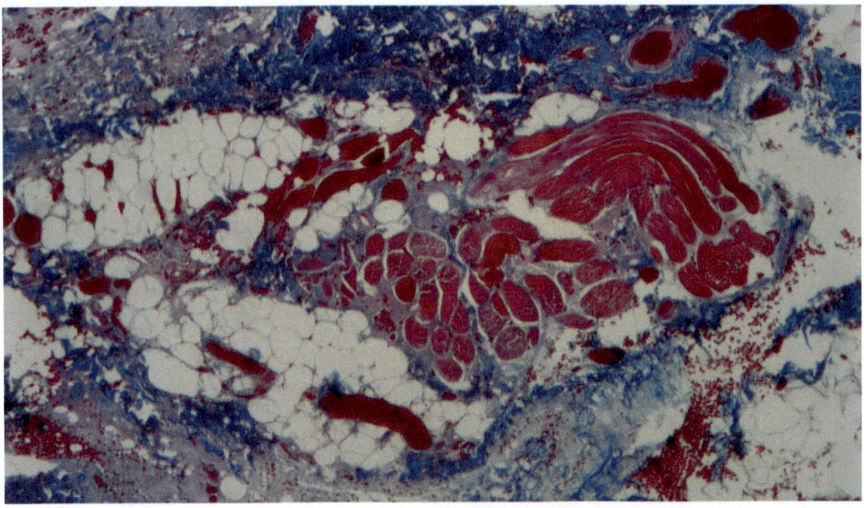

Fig. 5.8 Microphotograph of tissue excised from septum inguinalis. The large amount of muscle bundles highlighted show a wide range of damage in the center, ranging from hyaline (elongated and circular structures stained in red) to fibrotic degeneration (elongated and circular structures stained in pink). These degenerating muscle elements are surrounded by areas of fatty metaplasia of the myocytes (white circular elements). The connective tissue (colored in blue) shows evident edema with marked structural sufferance preluding degenerative disbanding. AM 50×

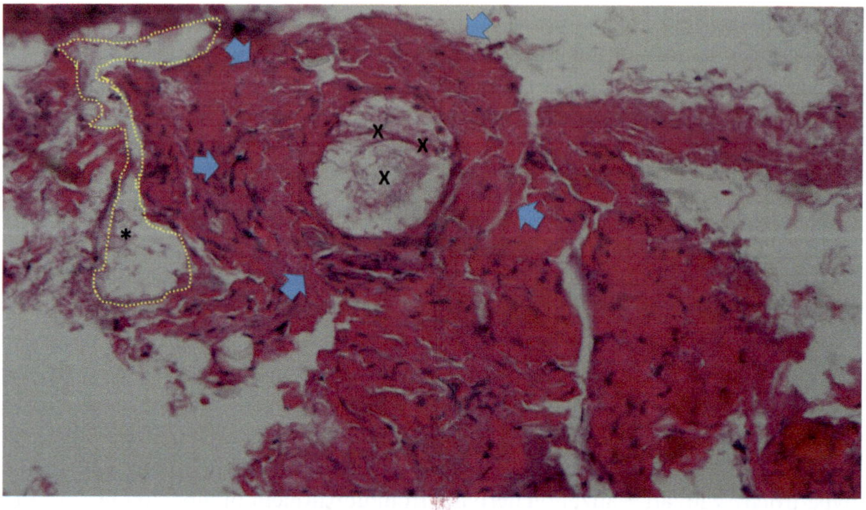

Fig. 5.9 Tissue specimen excised from the septum inguinalis in a patient with pantaloon hernia. Microphotograph highlights the inferior epigastric artery with severe hyperplasia of the tunica media (blue arrows). Structure of the muscular layer appears evidently altered by degenerative injury and incipient colliquation. Lumen of the artery is occupied by an organized thrombus (X) closely adherent to the vessel intima. Lateral to the artery, nearly unrecognizable, there is the inferior epigastric vein in a stage of advanced dissolution (yellow intermittent line). Lumen of the vein also contains a thrombotic element (*). Both vascular structures are surrounded by degenerated muscular bundles. EE 100×

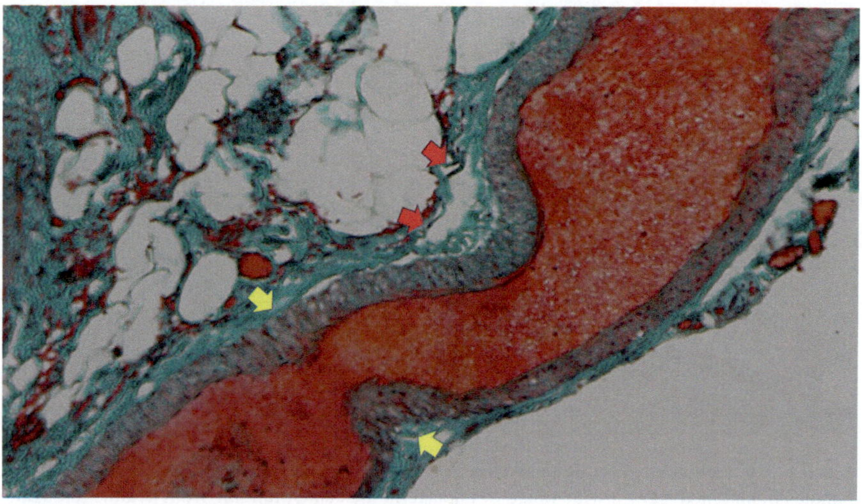

Fig. 5.10 Tissue specimen excised from the septum inguinalis in a case of pantaloon hernia. Mid-sized arterial structure with hyperplasia of the tunica media and noteworthy stenosis with approximately 70% reduction of the lumen (yellow arrows) caused by segmentary thickening of the muscular layer. Tunica adventitia (red arrows) is found in advanced degenerative disbanding preluding dissolution. Masson Trichrome 100×

5.5 Significance of Macro and Microscopic Findings Encountered in the Septum Inguinalis

The photographic sequence of the septum inguinalis highlighted in Figs. 5.3, 5.5, 5.6, and 5.7 demonstrate some significant, undeniable evidence: over time, the thickness of the muscular layers composing the anterior surface of the septum progressively reduce to complete disappearance. Analyses of these macroscopic alterations indicate that the anterior muscular layer of the septum is the first to suffer a degenerative insult that initially causes atrophy but subsequently continues until the complete disappearance of all muscle bundles covering the epigastric vessels. These macroscopic findings demonstrate that while the muscular damage involves the entire surface of the anterior aspect of the septum, the center of the septum that has no connection to the edges of the double ipsilateral hernias is even more involved. In particular, the muscular layers of the septum are progressively compressed against the robust inelastic fascia of the external oblique muscle until the typical damage of chronic compression develops. This means that muscular degeneration is not caused by expansion of the protrusions but rather by a degenerative insult deriving from another source. In this area, there is no other cause of degenerative damage barring the steady compression deriving from the orthostatic visceral impact. In effect, literature confirms that these muscular injuries are consistent with chronic

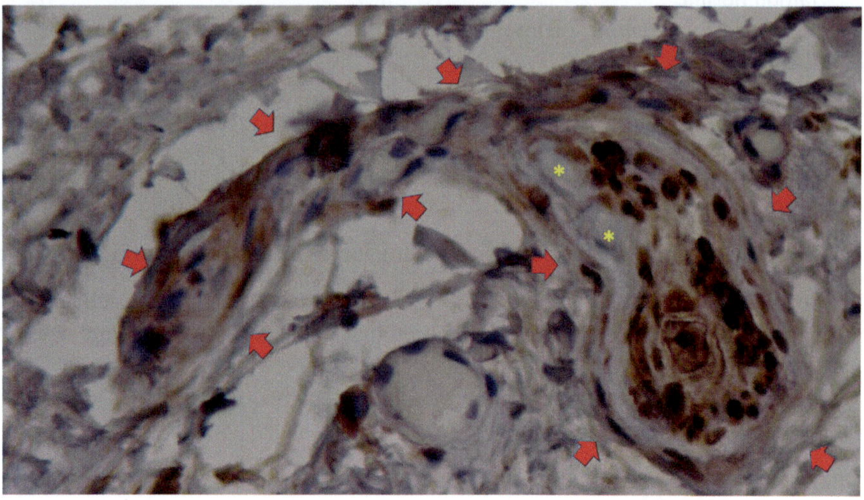

Fig. 5.11 Microphotograph of a biopsy sample excised from septum inguinalis. Elongated nerve structure (red arrows) with thickened myelin sheath showing fibrotic degeneration of the nerve axons (colored in pale brown). Some Schwann tubes appear empty (yellow asterisk) thus resembling a Wallerian degeneration. NSE400×

compressive damage [10–12]. The delicate muscular structures of the anterior surface are the first to suffer the effect of the degenerative damage, while the epigastric vessels are much more resistant: the solid multilayered structure protects the vessels for longer. However, persistent compressive insult over time continues and causes structural modifications to vessel architecture. The depicted vascular injuries, with associated negative effects on microcirculation and tissue metabolism, are considered a typical feature of chronic compressive damage [13–16]. An additional support for this explanation derives from the structural modifications seen in the nervous elements histologically detected within the septum inguinalis. Noteworthy thickening of the myelin sheath, fibrotic degeneration of the axons and sometimes also Wallerian degeneration that affect the nervous element are typical effects of chronic compressive damage [17–20].

5.6 Steady Orthostatic Visceral Impact Is Source of Inguinal Hernia Disease

The combined evidence deriving from the:

(a) Well-known gender-related differences of the pelvis shape.
(b) Macroscopic structural modifications encountered in the groin affected by pantaloon hernia.
(c) Structural worsening histologically verified in all tissue components of the groin.
(d) Progressive damage macroscopically highlighted and histologically confirmed in tissue components of the septum inguinalis.

Unquestionably direct the search for the pathogenetic roots of inguinal hernia to a single source:

the persistent impact of abdominal vector forces upon the inguinal backwall.

As portrayed in Figs. 5.12, 5.13, 5.14, 5.15, and 5.16, the etiological concept is strengthened by the undeniable consideration that the degenerative damage macro- and microscopically seen in the herniated groin can be triggered only by the sole source of compression in the lower anterior pelvis: steady orthostatic pressure of the abdominal viscera upon the groin.

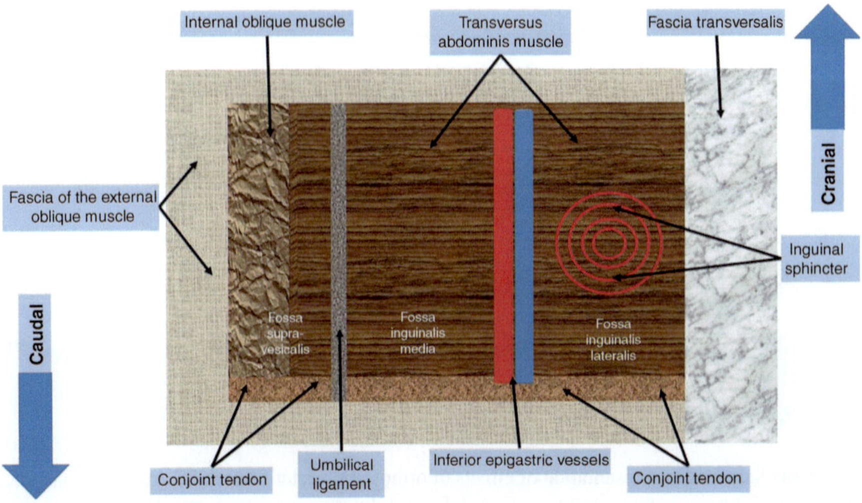

Fig. 5.12 Schematic representation of the structural layers which make up the septum inguinalis and neighboring anatomical elements (posterior, preperitoneal view)

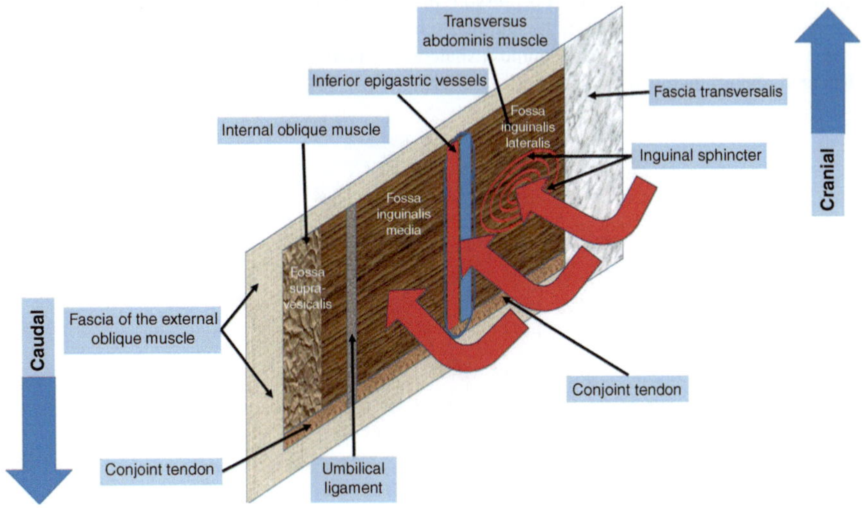

Fig. 5.13 Schematic representation of effects of orthostatic vector forces (red arrows) upon structures which make up the septum inguinalis (sagittal view). Initial stage: orthostatic pressure exerted by visceral content impacts a broad area of the inguinal backwall and specifically the zone between the lateral and the medial inguinal fossa, including the inferior epigastric vessels

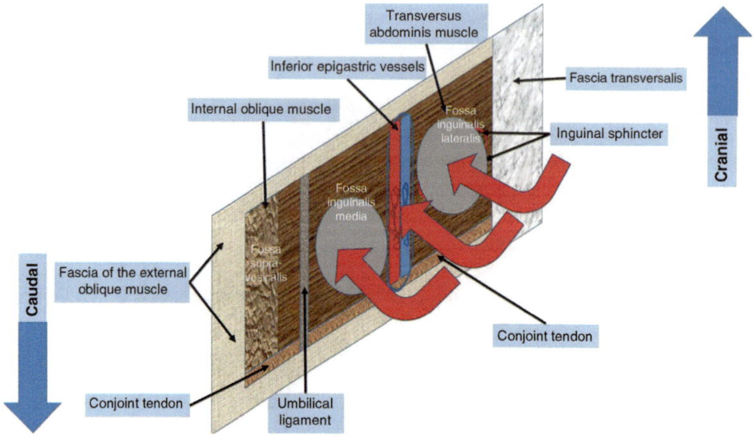

Fig. 5.14 Schematic representation of effects of orthostatic vector forces (red arrows) upon structures making up the septum inguinalis (sagittal view). Intermediate stage: steady orthostatic pressure of visceral vector forces worsens the metabolic processes of the musculature in the medial inguinal fossa and the inguinal sphincter. Muscular structure becomes atrophic and contractile function is impaired; the squeezing movement of the internal sphincter is compromised. Inferior epigastric vessels resist compressive effect with thickening of the tunica media and the adventitia. At the end of this the stage, visceral pressure disbands the muscular barrier and the abdominal content starts to protrude through the inguinal sphincter (indirect hernia) and the fossa inguinalis media (direct hernia), forming a double ipsilateral inguinal (pantaloon) hernia separated by the damaged septum inguinalis

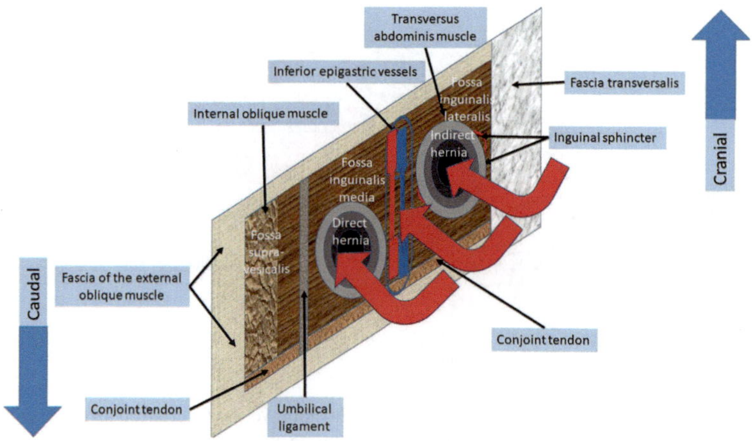

Fig. 5.15 Schematic representation of effects of orthostatic vector forces (red arrows) upon structures making up the septum inguinalis (sagittal view). Advanced stage: pantaloon hernia is finally established and pierces degenerated inguinal wall. The septum inguinalis is still protected by the epigastric vessels, which impede the impacting visceral forces; the structure of both vessels continues to deteriorate. Artery and arterial blood flows are markedly reduced by progressive hyperplasia of the tunica media that causes severe reduction of the lumen. Diminished blood flow further compromises vital metabolic functions of the perfused tissue. This further, irreversibly damages all tissue components of the inguinal wall. In the zone of impact, the vein is crushed, and venous blood outlet notably reduced. Venous segment close to the impact zone are ectasic and the neighboring tissue, flooded by edema, endures additional metabolic sufferance

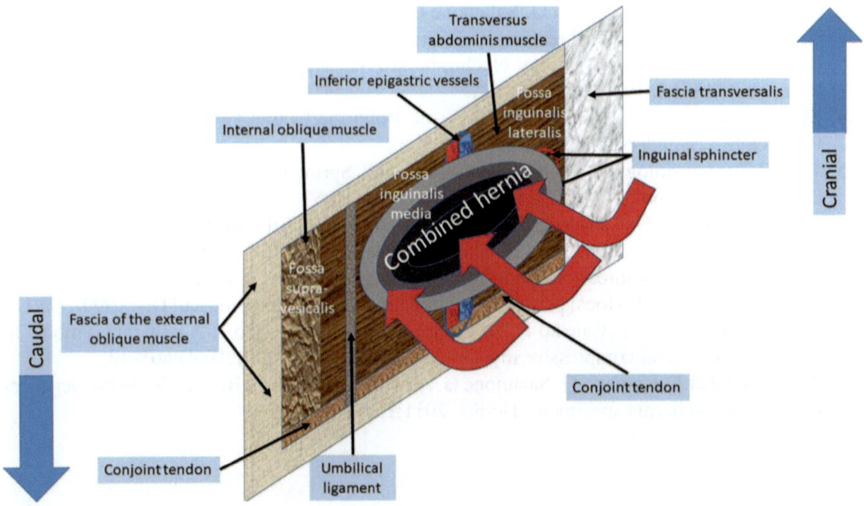

Fig. 5.16 Schematic representation of effects of orthostatic vector forces (red arrows) upon structures making up the septum inguinalis (sagittal view). Final stage: inferior epigastric vessels vanish under the destructive effect of visceral impact forces. The two hernias are unified constituting a single protrusion: the combined hernia

References

1. Amato G, Calò PG, Rodolico V, Puleio R, Agrusa A, Gulotta L, Gordini L, Romano G. The septum inguinalis: a clue to hernia genesis? J Investig Surg. 2018;31:1–9.
2. Ekberg O, Lasson A, Kesek P, Van Westen D. Ipsilateral multiple groin hernias. Surgery. 1994;115:557–62.
3. Woodward AM, Choe EU, Flint LM, Ferrara JJ. The incidence of secondary hernias diagnosed during laparoscopic total extraperitoneal inguinal herniorrhaphy. J Laparoendosc Adv Surg Tech A. 1998;8(1):33–8.
4. Kehlet H, Bay-Nielsen M. Nationwide quality improvement of groin hernia repair from the Danish Hernia Database of 87,840 patients from 1998 to 2005. Hernia. 2008;12:1.
5. Subhas G, Bakston D, Gupta A, Jacobs MJ, Mittal VK, Silapaswan S. Internal ring occlusion and floor and floor support: a novel technique for inguinal hernia mesh repair. Am Surg. 2010;76(9):933–7.
6. Amato G, Agrusa A, Romano G. Multiple ipsilateral inguinal hernias: more frequent than imagined, if undetected source of discomfort, pain, and re-interventions. Surg Technol Int. 2014;25:130–5.
7. Amato G, Agrusa A, Rodolico V, Puleio R, Di Buono G, Amodeo S, Gulotta E, Romano G. Combined inguinal hernia in the elderly. Portraying the progression of hernia disease. Int J Surg. 2016;(Suppl. 1):S20–9.
8. Hesselbach FK. Anatomisch-chirurgische Abhandlung über den Ursprung der Leistenbrüche. Würzburg: Baumgärtner; 1806.
9. Amato G, Agrusa A, Rodolico V, Caló PG, Puleio R, Romano G. Inguinal hernia: the destiny of the inferior epigastric vessels and the pathogenesis of the disease. Surg Technol Int. 2020;18:36.
10. Subhas G, Bakston D, Gupta A, Jacobs MJ, Mittal VK, Silapaswan S. Internal ring occlusion and floor support: a novel technique for inguinal hernia mesh repair. Am Surg. 2010;76(9):933–7.
11. Amato G, Agrusa A, Romano G, Salamone G, Gulotta G, Silvestri F, Bussani R. Muscle degeneration in inguinal hernia specimens. Hernia. 2012;16(3):327–31.

12. Amato G, Agrusa A, Romano G, Salamone G, Cocorullo G, Mularo SA, Marasa S, Gulotta G. Histological findings in direct inguinal hernia. Hernia. 2013;17(6):757–63.
13. Boyd GW. The patho-physiology of chronic arterial hypertension: a hypothesis. Clin Exp Pharmacol Physiol. 1980;7(5):541–4.
14. Kumar V, Abbas AK, Fausto N. Blood vessel. Robbins&Cotran Pathologic basis of disease. Philadelphia: Saunders; 2005. p. 513–5.
15. Tozzi P. The physiology of blood flow and artery wall. Springer editor, Sutureless Anastomoses, Darmstadt, Steinkopff 2007 12–24.
16. Amato G, Romano G, Salamone G, Agrusa A, Saladino VA, Silvestri F, Bussani R. Damage to the vascular structures in inguinal hernia specimens. Hernia. 2012;16:63–7.
17. Penkert G. Nerve compression syndrome-1. Chirurg. 1998;69:1114–22.
18. Kincaid JC. Stewart JD focal peripheral neuropathies. J Clin Neuromuscul Dis. 1999;1(2):113.
19. Kanchiku T, Taguchi T, Kaneko K, Yonemura H, Kawai S, Gondo T. A new rabbit model for the study on cervical compressive myelopathy. J Orthop Res. 2001;19(4):605–13.
20. Amato G, Ober E, Romano G, Salamone G, Agrusa A, Gulotta G, Bussani R. Nerve degeneration in inguinal hernia specimens. Hernia. 2011;15:53–8.

Chapter 6
New Aspects in the Functional Anatomy of the Groin

6.1 Introduction

Although the structural anatomy of the inguinal region is well defined, references concerning the functional anatomy of the inguinal structures are scanty in literature [1–6]. Indeed, the relationship between the anatomical elements forming the groin and the specific significance of these structures during the morphophysiological changes occurring during hernia formation has not been well defined. Only recently have specific histological studies, focused on the degenerative source of inguinal protrusion disease, contributed to better outlining the functional anatomy of the inguinal area [7–12]. Thus, the functional condition of the structures composing the herniated groin can finally be fully understood. It may therefore be said that for more than one century inguinal hernia repair techniques have been empirically carried out without understanding the real significance of the anatomical modifications that occur in the inguinal floor when a hernia protrusion is present. Lack of knowledge of the effective implications of these changes in the development of inguinal disease also contributed to mislabeling these pathological conditions. A typical example of this condition is the confusion there is in the classification of hernia protrusions; throughout the decades many different, and to some degree conflicting, versions have been proposed [13–17].

6.2 Morphology of the Inguinal Floor

The inguinal floor is a compound of different structures with specific morphological characteristics that vary depending on the visual perspective. In the anterior aspect (Fig. 6.1), covered by the fascia of the external oblique muscle, the main structures of the groin are:

G. Amato, *Inguinal Hernia: Pathophysiology and Genesis of the Disease*, https://doi.org/10.1007/978-3-030-95224-2_6

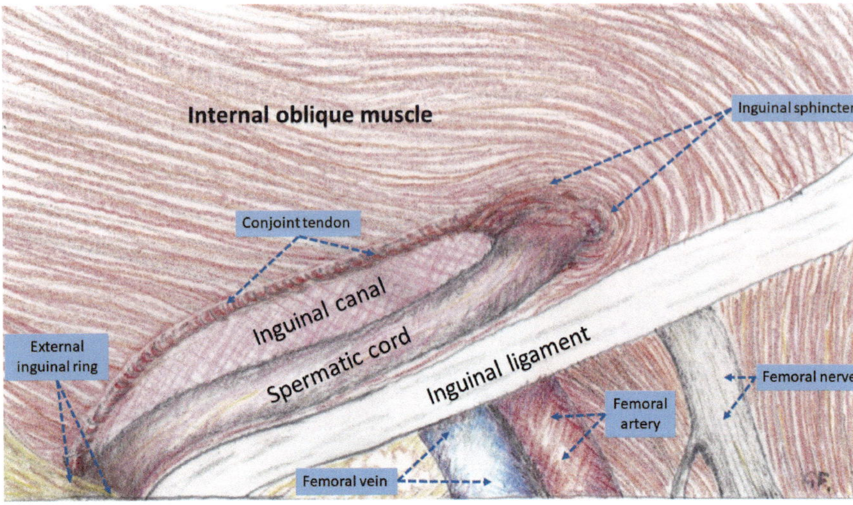

Fig. 6.1 The anterior aspect of the inguinal floor showing the main structures that compose this area © G. Ficile

- The inguinal canal, an anatomical pathway that contains the spermatic cord. It has two openings: the internal or inguinal sphincter, and the external inguinal ring that constitutes the exit route of the spermatic cord.
- The inguinal sphincter, a concentric muscular arrangement formed by interconnected fibers of the internal oblique and transversus abdominis muscle. It is the entrance of the spermatic cord to the inguinal canal.
- The spermatic cord, which contains the spermatic vessels and the ductus deferens. Enwrapped by the cremasteric muscle it enters from the inguinal sphincter, passes through the inguinal canal, and exits into the external inguinal ring.
- The internal oblique and the transversus abdominis muscles. In their distal boundary, they are joined together to form the conjoint tendon, which forms the cranial margin of the inguinal canal.
- The inguinal ligament that forms the lower margin of the inguinal canal.
- The external inguinal ring.

The posterior aspect (Fig. 6.2) is fully covered by the transversalis fascia; from medial to lateral it presents the following structures:

- The urachus, obliterated urinary conduct of the fetal period.
- The inguinal falx: This forms the lower medial portion of the conjoint tendon and is inserted in the pubic tubercle.
- The inguinal ligament: Obliterated remnant of fetal umbilical vessels.
- The inferior epigastric vessels that perpendicularly cross the inguinal backwall.
- The inguinal sphincter that forms the point where the testicular vessels and the ductus deferens become wrapped within the spermatic cord to cross the inguinal canal.

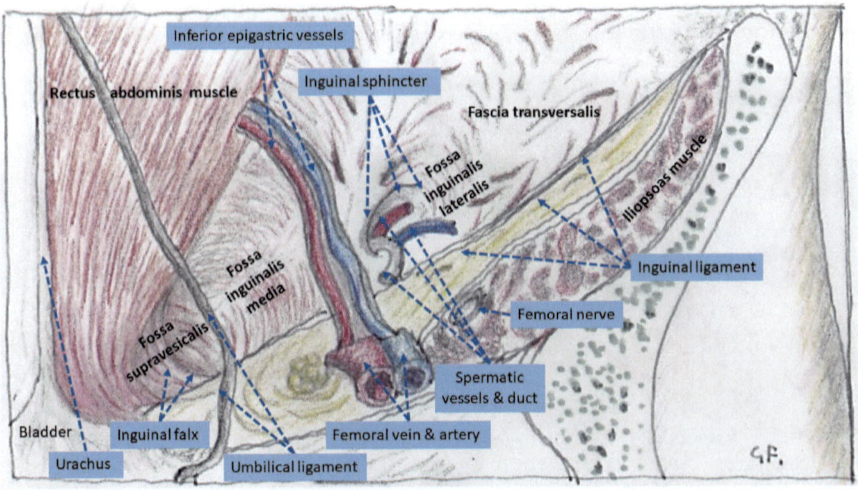

Fig. 6.2 Detailed structural composition of the posterior, preperitoneal surface of the groin. In the image, the three fossae constituting the inguinal backwall are represented: the supravesical, the medial, and the lateral. The backwall of the groin is covered by the fascia transversalis and longitudinally crossed by the urachus, the umbilical ligament as well as the inferior epigastric vessels. The spermatic vessels and the ductus deferens penetrate through the inguinal sphincter to form the spermatic cord. For clarity, the rectus muscle is depicted without its sheath

The inguinal area is also characterized by the presence of three fossae:

- The median or supravesical inguinal fossa bounded between the urachus and the umbilical ligament.
- The medial inguinal fossa between the umbilical ligament and the inferior epigastric vessels.
- The lateral inguinal fossa found laterally of the inferior epigastric vessels, containing the inguinal sphincter.

6.3 Hesselbach's Triangle: First Report in the Functional Anatomy of the Groin

The German anatomist and surgeon Franz Kaspar Hesselbach wrote the first description of this anatomical structure at the beginning of the nineteenth century [18]. He described a triangular-shaped anatomical component of the groin. The apex of Hesselbach's triangle is located in the pubic tubercle, the medial edge is formed by the lateral border of the rectus abdominis muscle while the inguinal ligament forms the lower boundary and the inferior epigastric vessels the lateral edge (Fig. 6.3).

Hesselbach described this anatomical structure to emphasize the concept that there is not one but two different types of inguinal hernia, each protruding from a different site of the inguinal floor, laterally and medially of the inferior epigastric

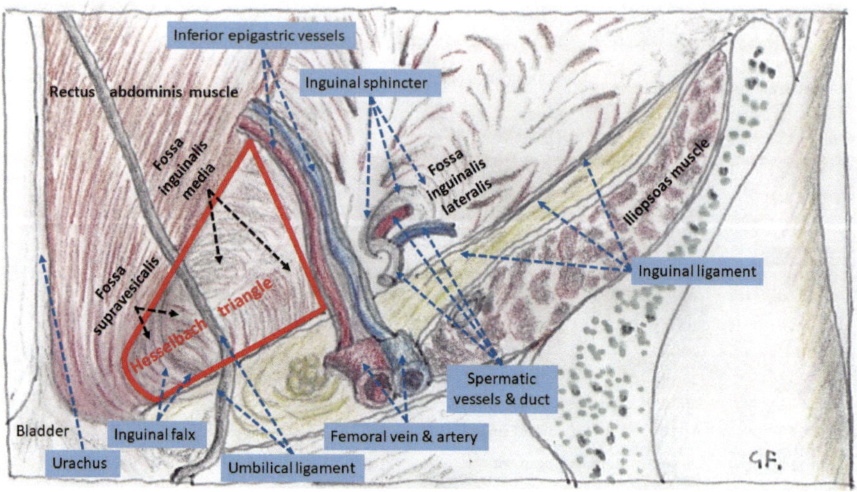

Fig. 6.3 Boundaries of Hesselbach's triangle (marked in red) and the concept of bipartition of the inguinal area. Medial margin of the triangle is formed by the rectus muscle (for clarity depicted without its sheath), inferior edge by the inguinal ligament, and lateral margin by the inferior epigastric vessels. Hesselbach's triangle comprises both the supravesical and the medial inguinal fossae and is also longitudinally crossed by the umbilical ligament. Lateral to the triangle there is the fossa inguinalis lateralis with the inguinal sphincter © G. Ficile

vessels. In modern times, these two types of hernia are referred to as indirect, arising from the inguinal sphincter (internal ring), and direct, which protrudes from the medial inguinal fossa. Therefore, it becomes obvious that in Hesselbach's description the inferior epigastric vessels played a fundamental role. Actually, Hesselbach simply divided the inguinal floor into two parts, lateral and medial of the epigastric vessels. These vascular structures served as a separation between the two types of hernia protrusions known at that time: direct and indirect hernias. However, by imagining only two inguinal areas, he did not understand that this district was functionally composed of three fossae, each bounded by a precise anatomical structure: the median/supravesical, medial, and lateral fossae. This is because Hesselbach underestimated the role of the umbilical ligament in delineating another important, although neglected part of the groin: the median compartment, also called supravesical fossa.

6.4 Critical Evaluation of Hesselbach's Functional Anatomy Concept Related to Inguinal Structures

The anatomical partition of the inguinal floor into two sections depicted by Hesselbach is a concept that resisted unaltered throughout two centuries. It was considered the main point of reference for almost all classification attempts of inguinal protrusions that for many decades simply contemplated only two types of hernia, direct and indirect hernias. However, updated knowledge deriving from recent studies on the anatomy of inguinal hernias allowed to highlight that this paradigm simply does not correspond to reality [6, 19, 20]. In fact, a simple observation of the anatomy of the posterior lower abdominal wall reveals that bipartition of this area does not seem congruent. The existence of an additional unknown element crossing this district has misled knowledge of the functional significance of the structures composing the groin: the umbilical ligament. Positioned between the pubic tubercle and the inferior epigastric vessels and remnant of fetal umbilical vessels, this ligamentous structure plays an important role and effectively helps in properly defining the functional anatomy of the groin. Unlike as imagined by Hesselbach, and disappointingly also by many surgeons in current years, not only do direct hernias protrude through Hesselbach's triangle, but also supravesical hernias. This is a neglected protrusion type penetrating the supravesical inguinal fossa medially of the umbilical ligament. Two types of supravesical hernias are described: the internal hernia that partially crosses the abdominal wall but remains restricted in the preperitoneal space and is normally diagnosed in the case of strangulation. The external type, more frequent than the previous, is often mistaken for a direct hernia [20]. This means that, in light of the above, Hesselbach's old-fashioned concept of functional anatomy is not only outdated but also inaccurate.

6.5 An Updated Concept of the Functional Anatomy of the Groin

Based on new findings from recent literature, the anatomy of the inguinal backwall should be characterized into three different components, each with a specific functional role (Fig. 6.4).

The tripartition of the inguinal floor is designed from the concept of the three anatomical fossae composing the inguinal area and consists of:

(a) A median, supravesical compartment corresponding to the fossa supravesicalis. It is a triangular-shaped segment of the inguinal backwall covered in its anterior aspect by the most distal inferomedial bundles of the internal oblique and the transversus abdominis muscles, often joined in the conjoint tendon. It is posteriorly found between the lateral margin of the rectus sheath, the inguinal falx, and the umbilical ligament. Similar to the other parts of the inguinal backwall, in the posterior surface it is covered by the transversalis fascia. By considering the Hesselbach bipartition, this site corresponds to the apex of the triangle and is where supravesical hernias (both internal and external types) develop [20].
(b) An intermediate compartment: This is caudally bounded by the inguinal ligament, medially by the umbilical ligament, and laterally by the septum inguinalis that separates the medial from the lateral fossa of the inguinal floor. In its anterior surface, it is covered by the muscle bundles of the internal oblique and transverse muscles merging together to form the conjoint tendon. Posteriorly, it

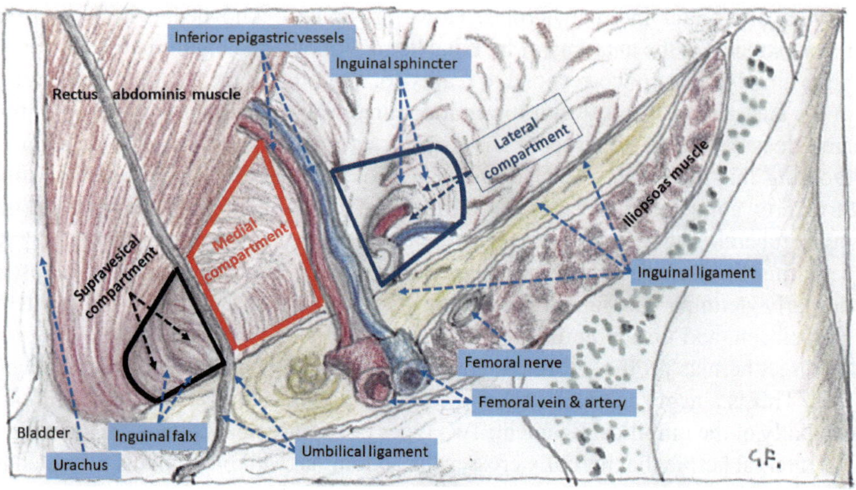

Fig. 6.4 The three compartments of the inguinal backwall. From medial to lateral: (a) supravesical (marked in black), is the site where the supravesical hernia protrudes; (b) the medial (marked in red), where the direct hernia arises; (c) the lateral inguinal fossa (marked in blue) is the site of indirect inguinal hernias. For clarity, the rectus muscle is depicted without its sheath © G. Ficile

is composed of the epigastric vessels and sheath. Containing more than just the inferior epigastric vessels, the septum inguinalis structure forms the lateral part of the medial inguinal fossa and the most medial margin of the inguinal sphincter. As in the rest of the inguinal floor, the transversalis fascia covers the preperitoneal surface of this compartment. This portion of the inguinal floor corresponds to the lateral portion of Hesselbach's triangle and is the site where direct inguinal hernias protrude.

(c) A lateral compartment that fully matches the lateral inguinal fossa and contains the inguinal sphincter composed of the interconnected fibers of the internal oblique and transversus abdominis muscles. From posterior to anterior it is crossed by the spermatic cord. This is the site where indirect inguinal hernias arise.

This subdivision of the anatomical components of the inguinal area is of great significance for an updated, detailed, and rational categorization of all types of inguinal hernias.

References

1. Casten DF. Functional anatomy of the groin area as related to the classification and treatment of groin hernias. Am J Surg. 1967;114(6):894–9.
2. Lytle WJ. Anatomy and function in hernia repair. Proc R Soc Med. 1961;54:967–70.
3. Bay-Nielsen M, Perkins FM, Kehlet H. Danish hernia database pain and functional impairment 1 year after inguinal herniorrhaphy: a nationwide questionnaire study. Am J Surg. 2001;233:1–7.

4. Amato G, Sciacchitano T, Bell SG, Romano G, Cocchiara G, Lo Monte AI, Romano M. Sphincter-like motion following mechanical dilation of the internal ring during indirect inguinal hernia procedure. Hernia. 2009;13:67–72.
5. Amato G, Marasa L, Sciacchitano T, Bell SG, Romano G, Gioviale MC, Lo Monte AI, Romano M. Histological findings of the internal inguinal ring in patients having indirect inguinal hernia. Hernia. 2009;13(3):259–62.
6. Amato G, Agrusa A, Rodolico V, Puleio R, Di Buono G, Amodeo S, Gulotta E, Romano G. Combined inguinal hernia in the elderly. Portraying the progression of hernia disease. Int J Surg. 2016;33(Suppl 1):S20–9.
7. Amato G, Ober E, Romano G, Salamone G, Agrusa A, Gulotta G, Bussani R. Nerve degeneration in inguinal hernia specimens. Hernia. 2011;15:53–8.
8. Amato G, Romano G, Salamone G, Agrusa A, Saladino VA, Silvestri F, Bussani R. Damage to the vascular structures in inguinal hernia specimens. Hernia. 2012;16:63–7.
9. Amato G, Agrusa A, Romano G, Salamone G, Gulotta G, Silvestri F, Bussani R. Muscle degeneration in inguinal hernia specimens. Hernia. 2012;16:327–31.
10. Amato G, Agrusa A, Romano G, Salamone G, Cocorullo G, Mularo SA, Marasa S, Gulotta G. Histological findings in direct inguinal hernia. Hernia. 2013;17:757–63.
11. Amato G, Calò PG, Rodolico V, Puleio R, Agrusa A, Gulotta L, Gordini L, Romano G. The septum Inguinalis: a clue to hernia genesis? J Investig Surg. 2018;31:1–9.
12. Amato G, Agrusa A, Rodolico V, Caló PG, Puleio R, Romano G. Inguinal hernia: the destiny of the inferior epigastric vessels and the pathogenesis of the disease. Surg Technol Int. 2020;36:pii: sti36/1274. [Epub ahead of print]
13. Nyhus LM, Klein MS, Rogers FB. Inguinal hernia. Curr Probl Surg. 1991;28:403–50.
14. Schumpelick V, Treutner KH, Arlt G. Classification of inguinal hernias. Chirurg. 1994;65:877–9.
15. Gilbert AI. An anatomic and functional classification for the diagnosis and treatment of inguinal hernia. Am J Surg. 1989;157:331–3.
16. Zollinger RM Jr. Classification systems for groin hernias. Surg Clin N Am. 2003;83:1053–63.
17. Miserez M, Alexandre JH, Campanelli G, Corcione F, Cuccurullo D, Pascual MH, Hoeferlin A, Kingsnorth AN, Mandala V, Palot JP, Schumpelick V, Simmermacher RKJ, Stoppa R, Flament JB. The European hernia society groin hernia classification: simple and easy to remember. Hernia. 2007;11(2):113–6.
18. Hesselbach FK. Anatomisch-chirurgische Abhandlung über den Ursprung der Leistenbrüche. Würzburg: Baumgärtner; 1806.
19. Amato G, Agrusa A, Romano G. Multiple ipsilateral inguinal hernias: more frequent than imagined, if undetected source of discomfort, pain, and re-interventions. Surg Technol Int. 2014;25:130–5.
20. Amato G, Romano G, Erdas E, Medas F, Gordini L, Podda F, Calò PG. External hernia of the supravesical fossa: rare or simply misidentified? Int J Surg. 2017;41:119–26.

Chapter 7
Classification of Inguinal Hernias Based on Functional Anatomy of the Groin

7.1 Introduction

Over the decades, several efforts have been made to achieve a shared concept in characterizing inguinal protrusions. Among these, an important role was played by the works of Casten, Gilbert, Nyhus, Zollinger, Schumpelick, and many other scientists [1–5]. The last attempt made by members of the European Hernia Society produced an additional classification with the intent to ease protrusion typing [6]. The need to categorize hernias arises from the responsibility of signing the operating register and clinical charts, apart from the duty of information toward patients and colleagues. Nevertheless, keeping in mind acronyms and/or numbers of all previous classifications is neither intuitive nor instinctive. This is one of the reasons why many surgeons have difficulty in classifying inguinal protrusions according to the aforementioned classifications, which in daily practice seem to be used only by a few experts but not by the majority of surgeons who deal with this frequent disease. Another issue to be stressed regards the lack or inadequate characterization of some hernia types, sometimes erroneously confused with other hernias or considered rare and, therefore, not included in many classification lists. It should also be noted that in the last decade, further evidence concerning pathogenesis of inguinal hernia as well as new studies on the functional anatomy of the groin have been brought to the attention of the surgical community. These investigations, highlighting progressive modifications of the functional anatomy of the inguinal floor when affected by hernia protrusion, hypothesize chronic visceral compression as the source of degenerative damage leading to inguinal hernia [7–11]. All these recent advances convey new contributions in defining modifications of the inguinal area affected by hernia. Therefore, a constructive evaluation of these findings may be helpful in better outlining inguinal protrusions.

G. Amato, *Inguinal Hernia: Pathophysiology and Genesis of the Disease*,
https://doi.org/10.1007/978-3-030-95224-2_7

7.2 Critical Revision of Inguinal Hernia Classifications

Following the latest updates concerning the functional anatomy of the groin, a critical review of the most used hernia classifications has been carried out. It is an endeavor to improve the effectiveness of tagging hernia protrusions by integrating evidence connected to the modification of the inguinal backwall. Aside from the differences between the single classification attempts, the revision is focused on defining the varieties of inguinal hernias by highlighting the peculiarity of each protrusion type in relation to the functional modifications that characterize the surgical anatomy of the herniated inguinal floor. In brief, the rationale of this work is to outline hernia types according to the location of the inguinal fossa/ae where the protrusion arises, i.e., the lateral, the medial, or the supravesical fossae. Listing the hernias by protrusion site also concerns defining the concomitant involvement of neighboring districts of the inguinal backwall. Hernias can either protrude in the form of multicomponent and confluent bulging, as seen in combined hernia, or as separate protrusions contextually arising from different sites of the same groin, the so-called multiple ipsilateral hernias [12]. No mention of dimension (volume) is given, since, to better define surgical strategy it is much more relevant to assess the site of the hernia defect and not the entire dimension of the protrusion (sac length and/or width). Therefore, it is sufficient to detail the location of the protrusion specifying whether it involves one or multiple components of the groin. This concept helps realize the size of the defect, which usually corresponds to the width of the fossa/ae where the hernia arises. Actually, with negligible differences of millimeters, the width of the fossa/ae is equivalent in all subjects [13, 14]. Photographic documentation provided herewith should further facilitate detailing specific hernia types.

7.3 Proposed Updated Classification Based on the Functional Anatomy of the Groin

To synoptically envisage the concept at the basis of the present critical revision, a table describing how the classification has been specifically conceived is presented (Table 7.1).

The first column of the list deals with the site of the inguinal backwall involved in the protrusion: it concerns single hernias affecting only one of the three fossae (the lateral, the medial, the supravesical). The last element of the first column regards multicomponent hernias, referred to as protrusions that arise through two or more fossae of the inguinal area. In the second column, the hernias are then grouped into primary or recurrent, definitions to be added to the specific hernia type: indirect, direct, supravesicalis, multicomponent, combined (confluent protrusions involving more than one fossa), or multiple ipsilateral. The third and last columns concern the description of each specific variant.

Table 7.1 Classification of inguinal hernias based on functional anatomy

Protrusion site	Hernia types: primary/ recurrent	Variants		
Lateral fossa—Inguinal sphincter	Indirect hernia	Pediatric/congenital hernia	Sportsman's hernia	Inguinoscrotal hernia
Fossa inguinalis media	Direct hernia			
Supravesical fossa	Hernia of the supravesical fossa	Internal	External	
Multicomponent	Combined bi-component	Supravesical + direct hernia	Direct + Indirect hernia	
	Combined tri-component	Supravesical+direct+indirect	Sliding hernia/Inguinoscrotal	
	Multiple Ipsilateral	Double or multiple indirect	Double or multiple Indirect+direct or/and supravesical	Triple: Indirect+direct+fossa supravesicalis

In detail, the initial three rows in the table indicate single protrusions. The first regards the protrusion that comes through the lateral fossa, the indirect hernia (Figs. 7.1 and 7.2) with its variants: pediatric/congenital, sportsman's (Fig. 7.3), and inguinoscrotal (Fig. 7.4). This type of large hernia descending into the scrotal sac can arise from the lateral fossa compartment alone without involving other components of the inguinal floor. This happens when the inguinal sphincter is thick enough

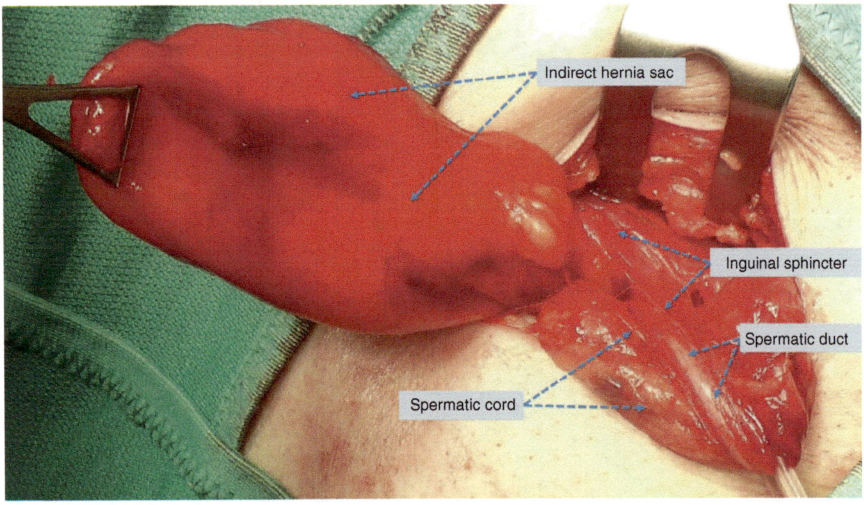

Fig. 7.1 Large obstructed indirect inguinal hernia protrusion arising from the inguinal sphincter

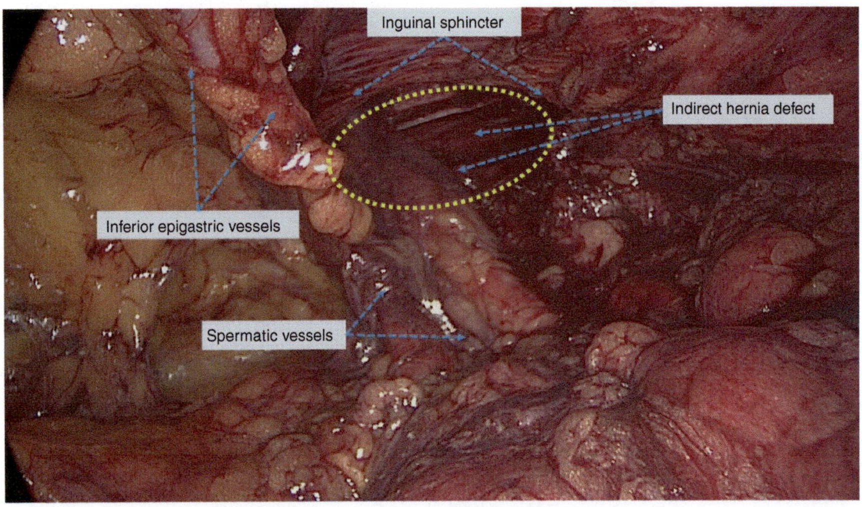

Fig. 7.2 Preperitoneal view in the frame of TAPP procedure showing an indirect inguinal hernia defect bounded by the inguinal sphincter

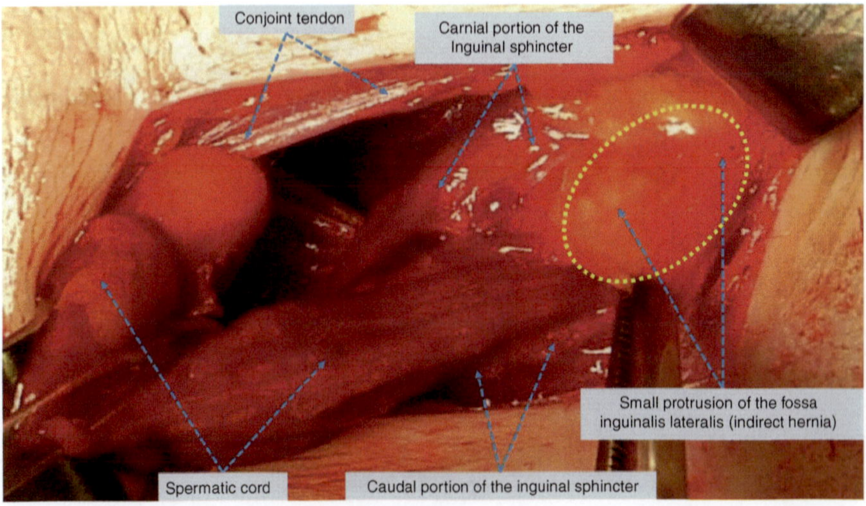

Fig. 7.3 Small indirect protrusion (yellow intermittent circle) arising from the internal ring in an active football player suffering from the typical symptoms of sportsman's hernia

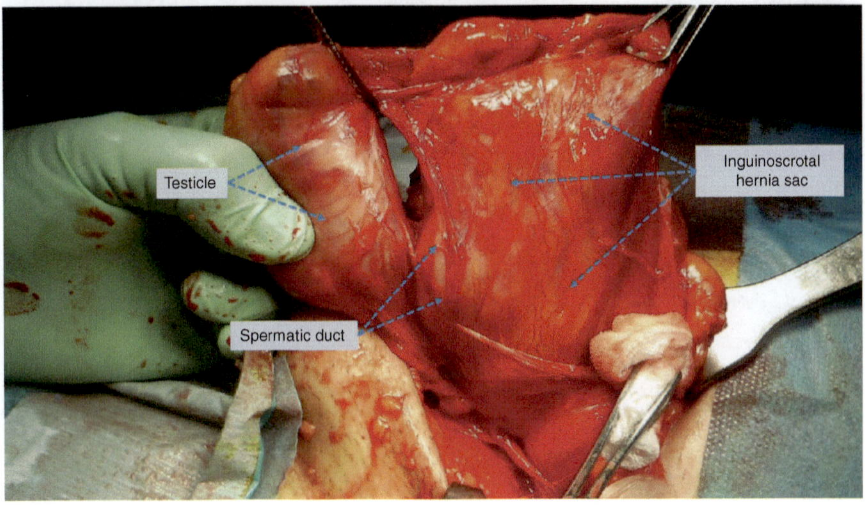

Fig. 7.4 Inguinoscrotal hernia. Sac of the protrusion has been partially separated from testicle. Spermatic duct is closely adherent to hernia sac

to constrain the hernia sac directed to the scrotum avoiding the involvement of the contiguous medial inguinal fossa.

In the second row, single protrusions involving only the medial inguinal fossa are referred to as direct hernia (Fig. 7.5). Nevertheless, unlike indirect hernia, a primary mono-component direct hernia alone never develops into an inguinoscrotal hernia, rather, if the protrusion in the medial fossa widens, it always involves more than one

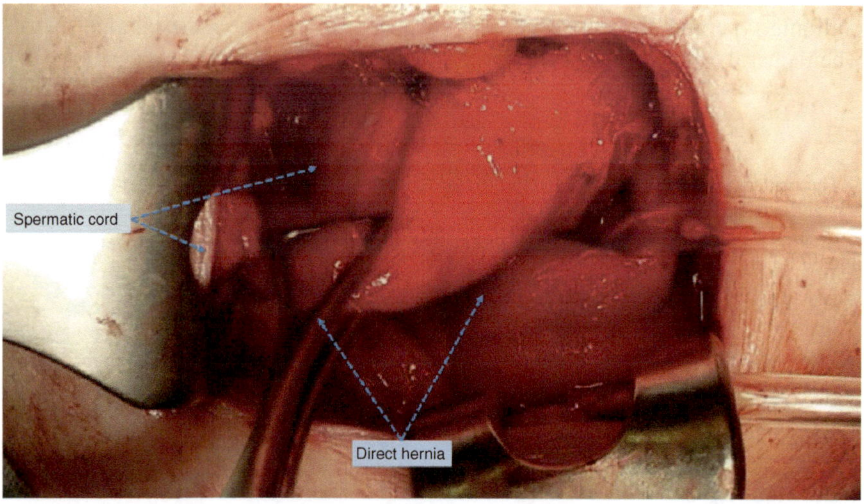

Fig. 7.5 Direct inguinal hernia arising from the medial inguinal fossa showing the typical bulging outline

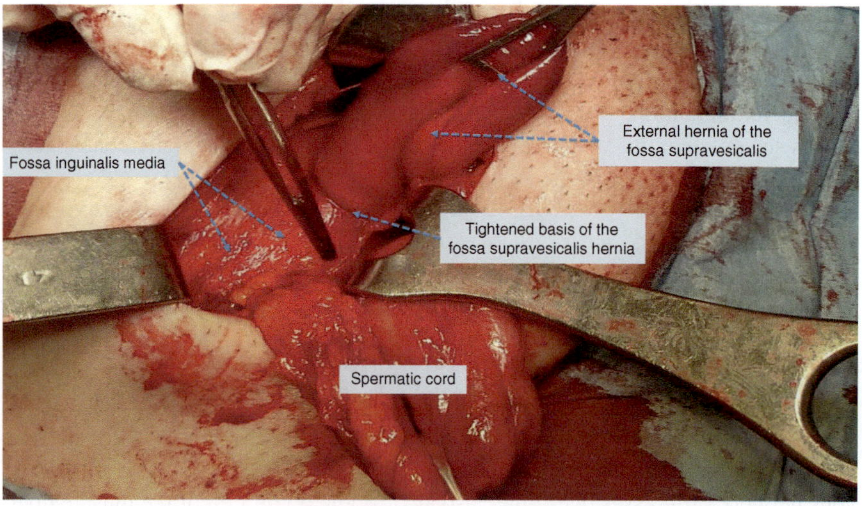

Fig. 7.6 External hernia of the supravesical fossa with its distinctive diverticular outline. The basis of the protrusion looks clearly tightened by a stricture that compresses the content

contiguous component of the inguinal floor before reaching the scrotum, constituting a specific, different type of protrusion: the combined hernia.

The third row of the table concerns hernias arising from the supravesical fossae that are divided into two subgroups: the internal and the external (Fig. 7.6). The internal variant of the supravesical protrusion is usually intraoperatively diagnosed in patients suffering acute intestinal obstruction. The external type, often mistaken for direct hernia and erroneously considered rare, shows a characteristic diverticular outline with a tightened basis. This particular aspect is caused by the rigid contour of the fossa made up of the hard, stiffened structures of the medial umbilical fold and the inguinal falx. This hernia type is known for a high tendency for incarceration and strangulation [15–17].

The subsequent, fourth row highlights the category of multicomponent hernias, which constitutes a group of protrusions that involve more than one component of the inguinal floor. The first subgroup of these hernias is made up of the bi-component combined hernia that is the result of the merging of two protrusions located in two neighboring fossae in one single unified protrusion. There are two types of these bi-component combined protrusions: one involving the most medial compartments of the inguinal floor, the supravesical and the medial inguinal fossae (Fig. 7.7). The second type of bi-component combined hernia involves the medial and the lateral inguinal fossae (Figs. 7.8 and 7.9).

The combined tri-component section characterizes a protrusion involving all three fossae converging into a single one and it is consequent to complete dissolution of the inguinal floor. This type is sub-grouped into tri-component combined (indirect + direct + fossa supravesicalis merging protrusions) (Fig. 7.10) and into sliding and/or inguinoscrotal hernia if the scrotal sac is occupied by the hernia (Figs. 7.4 and 7.11a, b).

Multiple ipsilateral hernias represent the last group of the list. They are made up of multiple independent protrusions concomitantly arising through one or more fossae separated from each other. These are subdivided into double or multiple indirect (Fig. 7.12) and double or multiple indirect + direct (Figs. 7.13–7.15).

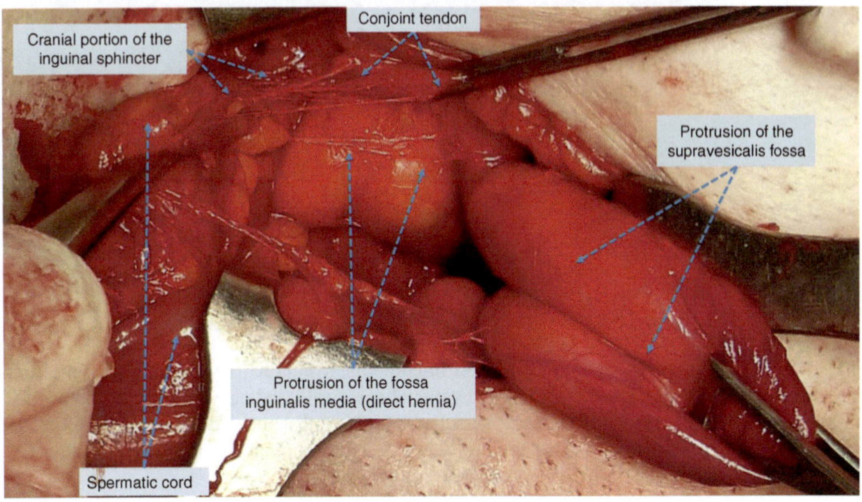

Fig. 7.7 Combined bi-component inguinal hernia made up of a protrusion of the fossa inguinalis media confluent to another protrusion of the fossa supravesicalis

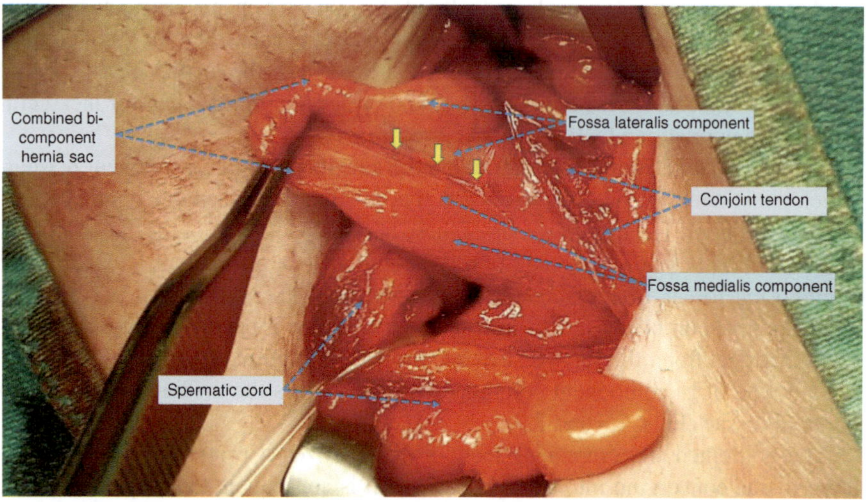

Fig. 7.8 Combined bi-component inguinal hernia involving the medial and lateral inguinal fossae (direct + indirect protrusions). The yellow arrows indicate the area of the already vanished inferior epigastric vessels

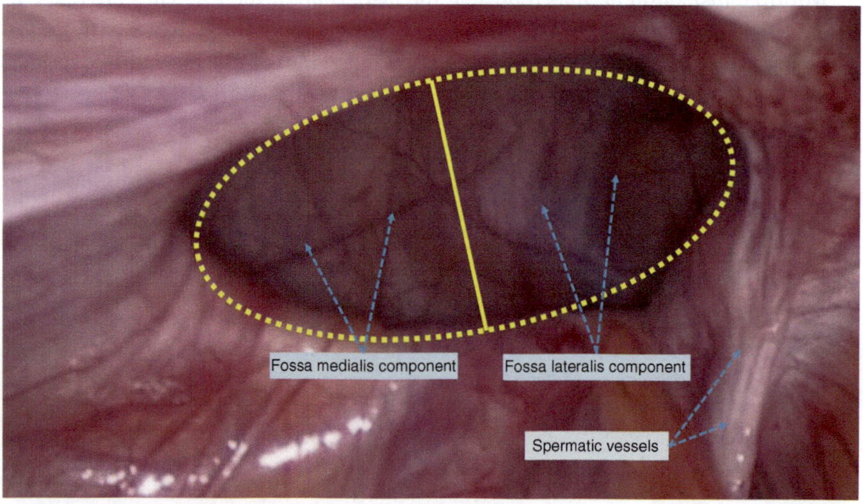

Fig. 7.9 Intra-abdominal view of combined bi-component inguinal hernia involving the fossa inguinalis media and the fossa lateralis. The yellow lines ideally indicate the limit of the two fossae. Of note, missing inferior epigastric vessels which have disappeared following degenerative damage caused by hernia disease. Spermatic vessels, seen through the transparency of the peritoneal sheath, have been laterally dislodged by hernia content

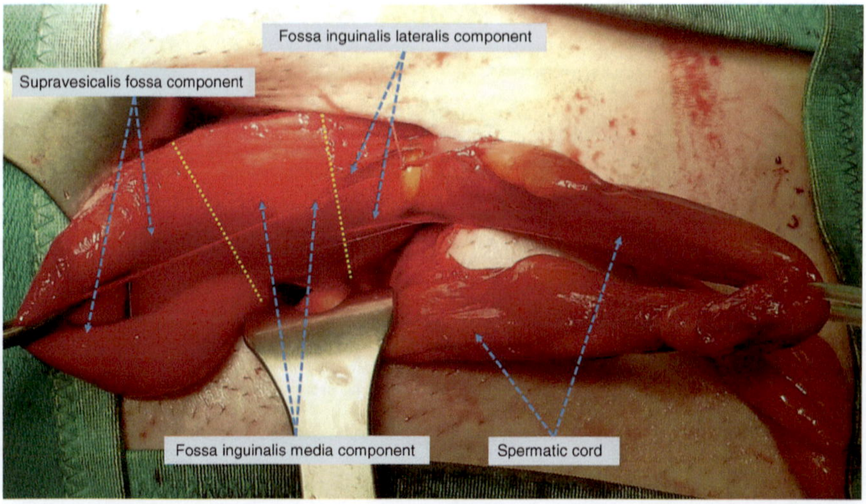

Fig. 7.10 Combined tri-component hernia, left. The intermittent yellow lines show each compartment making up the combined hernia: medially the typical diverticular-shaped protrusion of the fossa supravesicalis merges with a protrusion of the fossa inguinalis media that arrives at the lateral fossa and dislodges the spermatic cord sideways while entering the remains of the inguinal sphincter

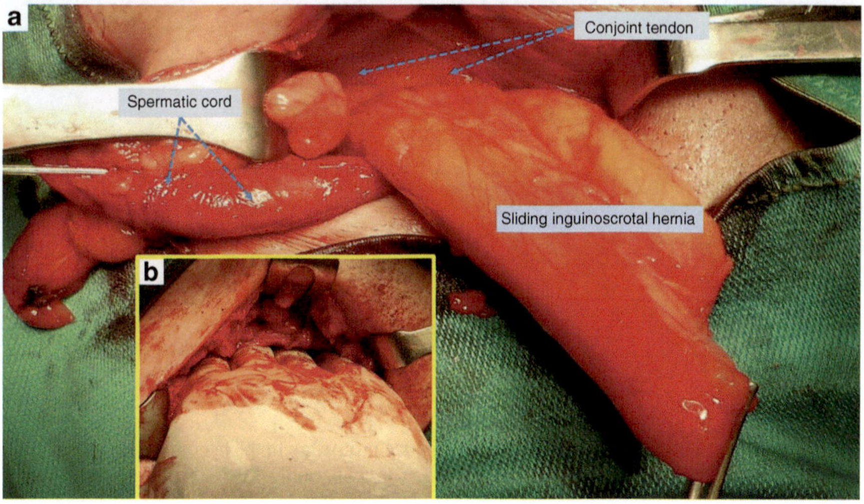

Fig. 7.11 (**a**): Typical sliding inguinoscrotal hernia of the right groin caused by the complete disbanding of the inguinal floor. (**b**) Fully degenerated inguinal floor allows returning the protrusion into the abdominal cavity by introducing four fingers beyond the abdominal wall into the preperitoneal space

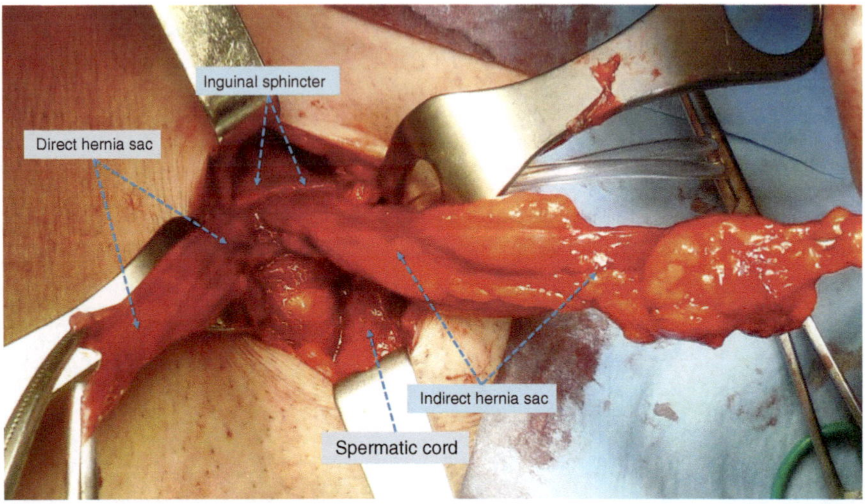

Fig. 7.12 Double ipsilateral inguinal hernia composed of two indirect protrusions arising through the inguinal sphincter

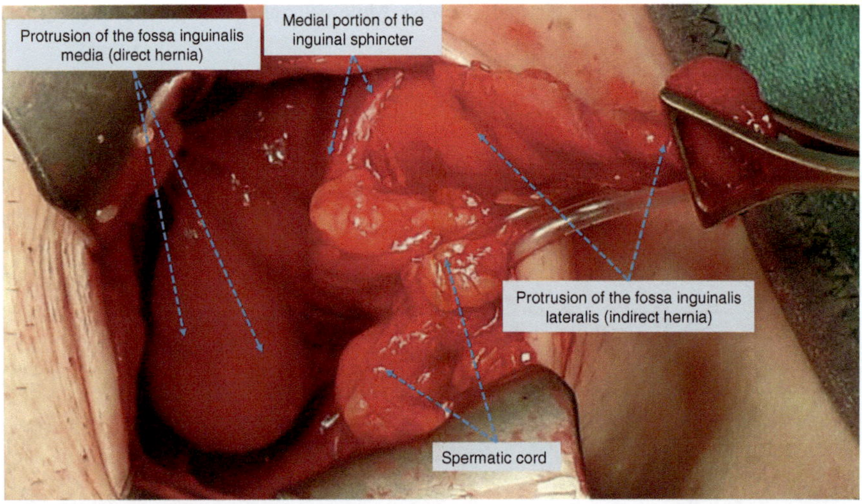

Fig. 7.13 Double ipsilateral hernia, left, showing one protrusion in the lateral inguinal fossa (indirect hernia) and one protrusion in the medial fossa (direct hernia)

It may also happen that the medial component of the multiple hernia is combined with a protrusion of the fossa supravesicalis hernia (Fig. 7.16). Another, rather infrequent, combination occurs when the double ipsilateral protrusion is formed by the concomitant presence of a separate direct hernia plus an external hernia of the supravesical fossa (Fig. 7.17).

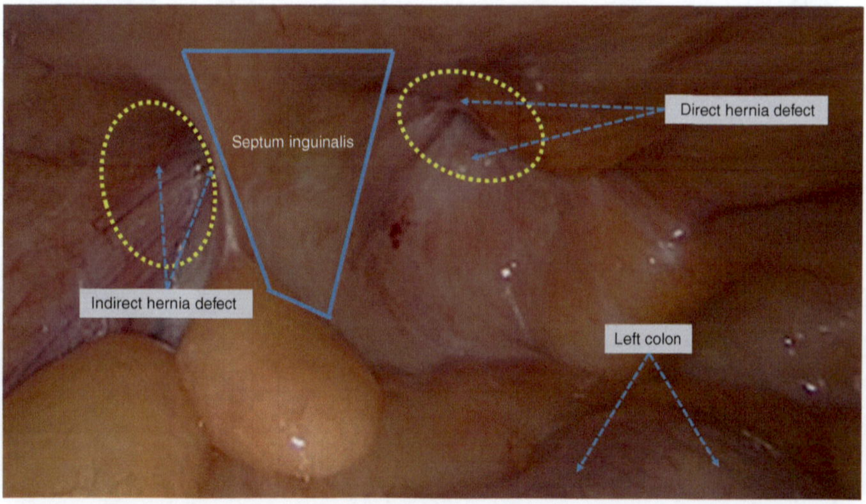

Fig. 7.14 Intra-abdominal view of left-sided double ipsilateral inguinal hernia composed of one defect of the medial inguinal fossa (direct hernia) and a defect in the lateral inguinal fossa (indirect hernia), both separated by the septum inguinalis

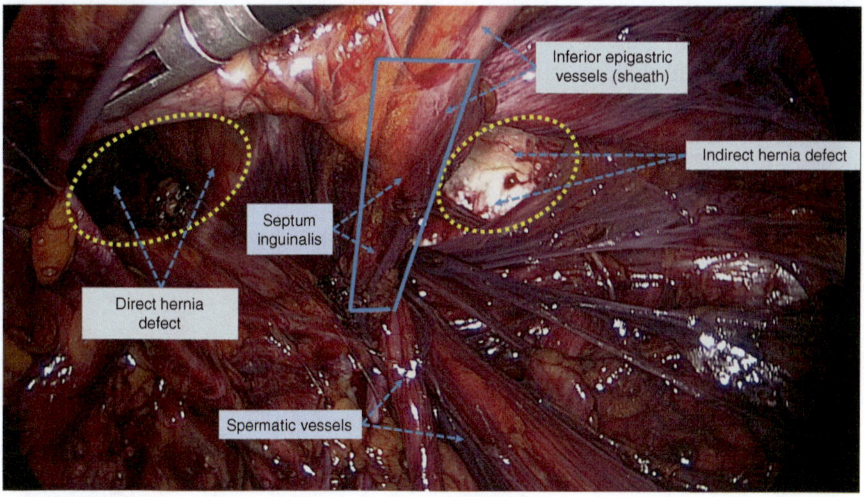

Fig. 7.15 Intraabdominal view of left-sided double ipsilateral inguinal hernia composed of one defect of the medial inguinal fossa and a defect of the lateral inguinal fossa, both separated by the septum inguinalis

A triple multiple ipsilateral hernia composed of three concomitant single protrusions occurring in each fossa and separated by a tissue septum has also been described and visually documented in literature [12]. It should be further stressed that the common occurrence of lipoma protruding from the preperitoneal space has

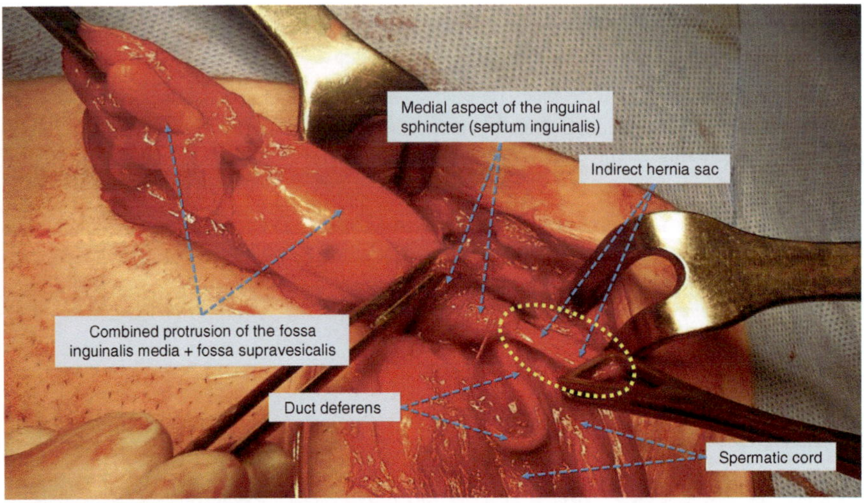

Fig. 7.16 Double ipsilateral hernia, left, showing a large, combined protrusion involving the medial and the supravesical inguinal fossae. Close to this combined hernia but separated by the medial aspect of the inguinal sphincter, a small indirect hernia (intermittent yellow circle) protrudes from the lateral inguinal fossa

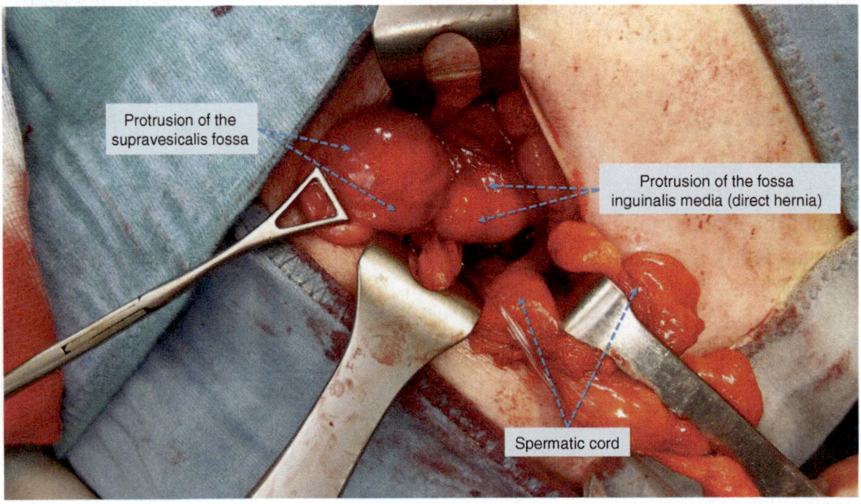

Fig. 7.17 Double ipsilateral inguinal hernia, left, composed of two separate protrusions: one emerging from the fossa supravesicalis and the second from the fossa inguinalis media

not been taken into consideration in the classification. These lipomatous extroflexions arising from the preperitoneal space outwardly cross the abdominal wall through the inguinal sphincter and almost exclusively accompany indirect hernias (Fig. 7.18).

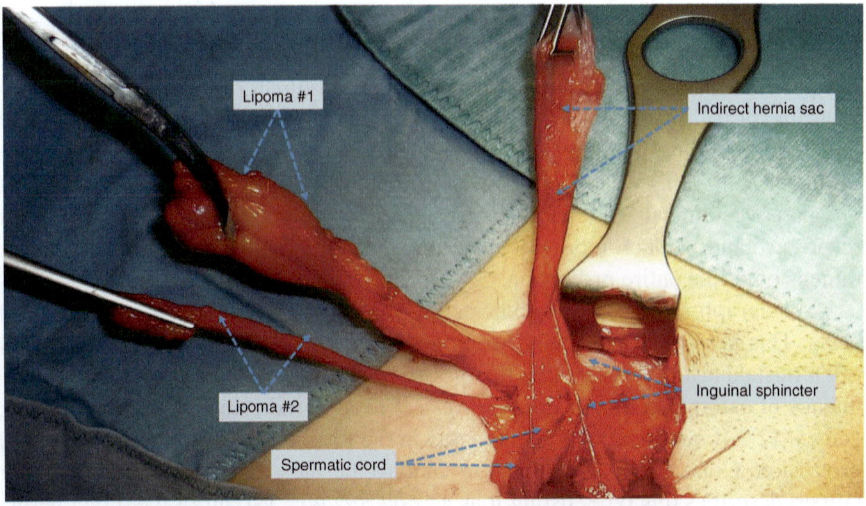

Fig. 7.18 Indirect inguinal hernia and two lipomas protruding from the inguinal sphincter

7.3.1 Do we Need another Hernia Classification List? Let us Explain this New One

The classification of inguinal hernia protrusions highlighted herewith aims to allow easy labelling of a hernia based on its location. The classifications currently used in hernia repair define the protrusion according to abbreviations and require a mnemonic endeavor that can lead to uncertainty. On the contrary, categorizing hernias by the site where they arise is simple and more accurate. Consequently, defining an indirect, direct, or combined hernia is spontaneous and incontestable.

An additional reason to move ahead with an updated classification emerges from the latest scientific evidence concerning the surgical anatomy of the groin [12, 15, 18]. In light of these recent reports, it would appear that the definition of some hernia types, such as combined, supravesical fossa and multiple ipsilateral hernias are insufficient, inadequate, or even lacking in many classification attempts.

For example, combined protrusions involving more than one fossa of the inguinal floor are reported in all classification attempts without mention of the fossae involved. This hernia type represents a typical disease of the third age [18] and recurs more frequently than others [19, 20]. To better understand the peculiarity of the combined hernia, we must keep in mind modifications of the functional anatomy of the inguinal area that, in these occurrences, assume a particular significance. Conventional gross anatomy of the groin describes the inguinal floor is composed of the deep inguinal ring laterally and Hesselbach's triangle medial to the epigastric vessels [21]. Nevertheless, as previously mentioned, functionally this concept may not be effective as the inguinal floor is functionally composed of three compartments: the supravesical, the medial, and the lateral [22]. Following this model, it becomes easy to categorize combined hernias by specifying the fossae where the hernia protrudes. This allows detailing confluent/combined protrusions as bi-component (and specifically the variants, direct + indirect or direct + fossa supravesicalis) or tri-component, when all three fossae are involved. This is fundamental in determining the site of the hernia defect and above all the diameter, which can be estimated with a high degree of precision by ultrasound or CT [23]. This kind of preoperative clinical evaluation is considered an important predictive factor of recurrence and is much more effective than the empirical concept of assessing the dimension of the entire protrusion.

A paragraph apart must be dedicated to the external hernia of the supravesical fossa. This hernia type has long been considered rare [17], probably because it is often mistaken for direct hernia: this has been proven wrong [15]. In fact, the frequency of external hernia of the supravesical fossa is indicated at ca. 5%, if single, and ca. 12% if confluent to a direct hernia in the form of a bi-component combined protrusion. Concerning categorization, among the most used classifications, only Gilbert describes this type, listing it as a *"diverticular"* variant of the direct hernia [4]. Apparently, no other meaningful classification registers this hernia type as an autonomous entity. The almost neglected acknowledgment of this intriguing protrusion type, which shows a high tendency to strangulation, makes its meticulous detection mandatory [16].

Another group of protrusions that have been totally ignored in all previous classification lists concerns multiple ipsilateral hernias, represented by more than one protrusion separately arising from the same groin. Honestly, it is hard to understand why this cohort of protrusions has not been taken into consideration in the past, despite frequency being estimated at ca. 10% of all hernias [12]. In light of this evidence, it would seem undisputable that this hernia category should not be considered a rarity but a well-represented group, worthy of being defined and detailed in all its configurations. In the classification presented above, these multiple hernias are listed, highlighting all possible arrangements. The spectrum of combinations varies from multiple independent separate protrusions of the lateral fossa (the most frequent occurrence) to the combination of one or more indirect hernia protrusions contextually present in the same groin together with a direct hernia. Or, one direct hernia plus another protrusion arising separately from the supravesical fossa. Regarding the latter, it is suggested to avoid using the term pantaloon hernia, since this classifies a double protrusion classically related to a direct and indirect protrusion of similar dimensions, resembling two legs of a pair of pants. Double ipsilateral hernias are often formed by protrusions of different dimensions, e.g., one small plus one larger, therefore, it appears obvious that the term pantaloon hernia is, in the vast majority of cases, misleading (Fig. 7.12).

7.4 Accurate Intraoperative Classification of Inguinal Hernia May Improve Surgical Treatment Results

Classifying inguinal hernias during repair procedures is an important duty of the surgeon. It implies choosing the adequate surgical approach, if necessary tailored for each specific case. Exact intraoperative definitions of abdominal protrusions are also beneficial to colleagues that may have to manage a recurrence. For this reason, the surgical community should envision a definite description of the protrusion type encountered as mandatory, even better if documented with images. In the past years, there has not been enough attention paid to this issue but complying with this simple task can also be helpful for patients. In this regard, it should be stressed that the involvement of more than two fossae suggests an increased risk of recurrence, therefore, this constitutes an important factor that should be taken into consideration for an adequate surgical strategy aiming to avoid intra- and postoperative complications. Furthermore, if when repairing a recurrent hernia, the site (not the dimension) of the previously managed hernia is unknown, it would be a real challenge to intraoperatively categorize the hernia as a real recurrence of the previously repaired protrusion. In brief, it cannot be ascertained if the second protrusion is a real recurrence or a new hernia protruding from a different site from the already repaired hernia. Alternatively, as hypothesized in literature, the forgotten hernia, namely the additional ipsilateral protrusion that went undetected during the first repair should be taken into account [12]. In these cases, the correct characterization of the primary hernia surely makes the difference.

Summarizing, inguinal hernia should be categorized by describing the site of the defect not the dimension of the entire protrusion. In the case of combined hernia, the involved fossae should be indicated exactly. This procedural behavior also implies a meticulous search for multiple ipsilateral protrusions. This helps detect hidden inguinal protrusions concealed by adhesion bridles or fat tissue. It would be useful, if contextually present, to document these particular hernias with images when possible. In accordance with these principles, releasing photographic documentation of the surgical procedure is recommended when discharging the patient.

References

1. Casten DF. Functional anatomy of the groin area as related to the classification and treatment of groin hernias. Am J Surg. 1967;114:894–9.
2. Nyhus LM, Klein MS, Rogers FB. Inguinal hernia. Curr Probl Surg. 1991;28:403–50.
3. Schumpelick V, Treutner KH, Arlt G. Classification of inguinal hernias. Chirurg. 1994;65:877–9.
4. Gilbert AI. An anatomic and functional classification for the diagnosis and treatment of inguinal hernia. Am J Surg. 1989;157:331–3.
5. Zollinger RM Jr. Classification systems for groin hernias. Surg Clin N Am. 2003;83:1053–63.

6. Miserez M, Alexandre JH, Campanelli G, Corcione F, Cuccurullo D, Pascual MH, Hoeferlin A, Kingsnorth AN, Mandalà V, Palot JP, Schumpelick V, Simmermacher RK, Stoppa R, Flament JB. The European Hernia Society groin hernia classification: simple and easy to remember. Hernia. 2007;11(2):113–6.
7. Amato G, Marasa L, Sciacchitano T, Bell SG, Romano G, Gioviale MC, Lo Monte AI, Romano M. Histological findings of the internal inguinal ring in patients having indirect inguinal hernia. Hernia. 2009;13(3):259–62.
8. Amato G, Ober E, Romano G, Salamone G, Agrusa A, Gulotta G, Bussani R. Nerve degeneration in inguinal hernia specimens. Hernia. 2011;15:53–8.
9. Amato G, Romano G, Salamone G, Agrusa A, Saladino VA, Silvestri F, Bussani R. Damage to the vascular structures in inguinal hernia specimens. Hernia. 2012;16:63–7.
10. Amato G, Agrusa A, Romano G, Salamone G, Gulotta G, Silvestri F, Bussani R. Muscle degeneration in inguinal hernia specimens. Hernia. 2012;16(3):327–31.
11. Amato G, Agrusa A, Romano G, Salamone G, Cocorullo G, Mularo SA, Marasa S, Gulotta G. Histological findings in direct inguinal hernia. Hernia. 2013;17(6):757–63.
12. Amato G, Agrusa A, Romano G. Multiple ipsilateral inguinal hernias: more frequent than imagined, if undetected source of discomfort, pain, and re-interventions. Surg Technol Int. 2014;25:130–5.
13. Rabe R, Yacapin CPR, Buckley BS, Macario Faylona J. Repeated in vivo inguinal measurements to estimate a single optimal mesh size for inguinal herniorrhaphy. BMC Surg. 2012;12:19.
14. Diana G, Arcara M, Guercio G, Sommariva V, Peri G, Farina F, Marcianò V, Ridola C. Anatomical and clinical aspects of inguinal canal, during inguinal hernia. Surg Radiol Anat. 1995;17:209.
15. Amato G, Romano G, Erdas E, Medas F, Gordini L, Podda F, Calo PG. External hernia of the supravesical fossa: rare or simply misidentified? Int J Surg. 2017;41:119–26.
16. Sozen I, Nobel J. Inguinal mass due to an external supravesical hernia and acute abdomen due to an internal supravesical hernia: a case report and review of the literature. Hernia. 2004;8:389–92.
17. Ekberg O, Lasson A, Kesek P, Van Westen D. Ipsilateral multiple groin hernias. Surgery. 1994;115:557–62.
18. Amato G, Agrusa A, Rodolico V, Puleio R, Di Buono G, Amodeo S, Gulotta E, Romano G. Combined inguinal hernia in the elderly. Portraying the progression of hernia disease. Int J Surg. 2016;33(Suppl 1):S20–9.
19. Burcharth J, Andresen K, Pommergaard HC, Bisgaard T, Rosenberg J. Recurrence patterns of direct and indirect inguinal hernias in a nationwide population in Denmark. Surgery. 2014;155(1):173–7.
20. Burcharth J, Pommergaard HC, Bisgaard T, Rosenberg J. Patient-related risk factors for recurrence after inguinal hernia repair: a systematic review and meta-analysis of observational studies. Surg Innov. 2015;22(3):303–17.
21. Hesselbach FK. Anatomisch-chirurgische Abhandlung über den Ursprung der Leistenbrüche. Würzburg: Baumgärtner; 1806.
22. Amato G, Calò PG, Rodolico V, Puleio R, Agrusa A, Gulotta L, Gordini L, Romano G. The septum inguinalis: a clue to hernia genesis? J Investig Surg. 2020;33(3):231–9.
23. Picasso R, Pistoia F, Zaottini F, Airaldi S, Miguel Perez M, Pansecchi M, Tovt L, Sanguinetti S, Möller I, Bruns A, Martinoli C. High-resolution ultrasound of spigelian and groin hernias: a closer look at fascial architecture and aponeurotic passageways. J Ultrason. 2021;21(84):53–62.

Chapter 8
State of the Art and Future Perspectives in Inguinal Hernia Repair

8.1 State of the Art in the Treatment of Inguinal Hernia

Despite its frequency, a wide range of postoperative complications affects the management of inguinal hernia, which can only be resolved surgically. Historically, different types of surgical procedures have been proposed over the years. In the modern era, for a very long period Prof. Bassini's method was the most used technique all over the world [1]. The use of this surgical technique, together with other comparable variants referred to as pure tissue repair procedures, spanned two centuries, until present times [2, 3]. Only in the 1960s did a new concept of cure start to spread [4]. It concerns the deployment of a flat mesh over the hernia defect to reinforce the groin thanks to fibrotic apposition in the mesh (Fig. 8.1) [5–7].

This surgical approach contributed to the dramatic decrease in the rate of recurrence, but on the other hand allowed the development of specific complications caused by both the prosthetic material and the surgical technique itself [8]. The concept of reinforcing the groin with the apposition of a mesh of synthetic biocompatible material, mostly made of polypropylene, has also been borrowed in

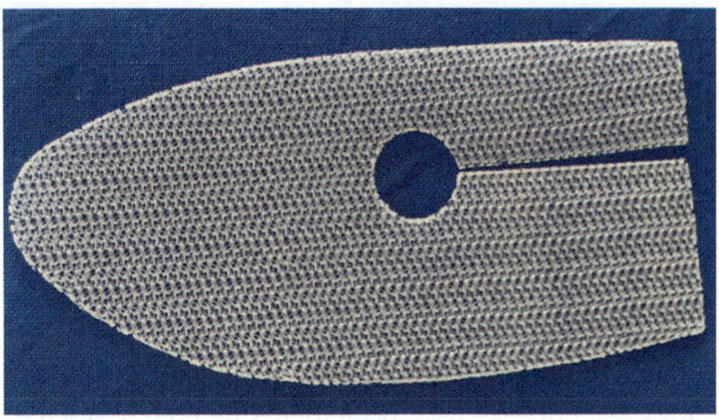

Fig. 8.1 A conventional pre-shaped polypropylene flat mesh for open anterior inguinal hernia repair

G. Amato, *Inguinal Hernia: Pathophysiology and Genesis of the Disease*,
https://doi.org/10.1007/978-3-030-95224-2_8

laparoscopic inguinal hernia repair, which in the last decade has been increasingly performed compared to the conventional anterior open technique [9]. Uncontrolled stiff fibrotic scar plate as a biologic response and the need for fixation of the mesh are the main issues of this treatment concept. Discomfort, long-lasting pain, tissue tear, and hematomas are the most complained about postoperative complications of the surgical procedure [9–14]. However, despite the source of these frequent postoperative adverse events being well identified, the significance of the complications has not been adequately perceived and, therefore, no effective solution has been found to resolve the problems. All these adverse events are simply the consequence of a discrepancy between the physical attitude of the prosthetics and the physiological features of the recipient. More in detail, it concerns the static, passive behavior of the mesh compared to the highly mobile aspect of the groin. This discrepancy is then further amplified by mesh fixation, which is needed to avoid dislodgement of the implant. In light of the above, it is evident that the current solutions for inguinal hernia disease have been developed without paying attention to the specific physiology of the inguinal area. Actually, using static, fixated implants to resolve a disease in one of the most motile districts of the body is logically unphysiological. Furthermore, if an analysis focused on the pathogenesis of the disease and the effects of the treatment is made, both the surgical techniques and the prosthetics used to turn out to be completely incongruent to resolve the pathology at its roots. By considering the degenerative genesis of inguinal hernia, it is evident that the disease can only be resolved by stopping degeneration and activating the regeneration of the vanished tissue. However, the stiff fibrotic scar plate of flat meshes does not correspond to regeneration; it is, rather, a common foreign body response. In the delicate inguinal area, uncontrolled fibrotic proliferation around the mesh can lead to enveloping or compression of the highly sensitive nervous structures running along the inguinal canal. This phenomenon is the basis of the frequent and most feared unpleasant complication after conventional inguinal hernia repair: chronic pain, a never-ending painful syndrome that altogether upsets patients' quality of life [15–17].

8.2 Is Overcoming the Incongruences of the Currently Available Concept of Cure Possible?

By analyzing the state of the art in the treatment of inguinal hernia, it is clear that for more than a century, neither the basic physiology nor the pathogenesis of the disease has been considered in the development of surgical techniques for the care of the herniated groin. Surprisingly, if a consideration is made on how many renowned scientists have been involved in the search for an effective solution to inguinal protrusions one remains astonished at how these simple concepts of physiology and etiology have been totally ignored. Even the frequently occurring adverse events for decades were not perceived as an alarm bell: the search to improve treatment results repeatedly came to a dead end.

Only recently has a different line of thought found an exit route to the old-fashioned, controversial model of cure that for more than half a century continued to be acritically utilized in inguinal hernia patients. An updated therapy concept deriving from new evidence in the physiology and functional anatomy of this complex part of the body, in addition to the latest findings on the pathogenesis of inguinal protrusions allowed an opening to a new pathway for a more physiological and pathogenetically coherent principle of cure of this intriguing disease [18–24].

8.3 A New Advanced Vision for the Treatment of Inguinal Hernia

Considering the particular physio-morphological characteristics of the groin and the specificity of the degenerative source of inguinal hernia, the conventional old-fashioned model of therapy based on a simple static flat mesh deployed over the defect appears to no longer meet the needs for resolving the multifaceted aspects of the disease. Instead, the ideal model of cure should utilize tools able to cope with the natural dynamic cyclical load of the inguinal musculature in a more physiological fashion. This new model of treatment should also be based on an innovative kind of device, which unlike the poor-quality biologic response of flat meshes should induce a fully congruent regeneration of the structures composing the inguinal barrier.

In addition to these noteworthy features, this newly envisioned therapeutic tool should achieve the following important specifics:

(a) Avoid any kind of limitation or impairment of inguinal movements, as occurs with conventional prosthetics fixated with sutures, tacks, or glue to the myotendineal structure of the groin.
(b) Strive for full, permanent obliteration of the hernia defect.

To fulfill these expectations, a series of translational studies involving physiology, pathology, histology, anatomy, prosthetic material science, and bioengineering was initiated at the beginning of the current century to outline a new method for the cure of inguinal hernia. A working theory involved using the same polypropylene material as conventional implants but modifying the outline into a 3D shape with inherent springiness and intrinsic memory. The hypothesis at the basis of these attempts involved designing a 3D structure able to confer the dynamic responsivity required to turn the biologic response into a probiotic, regenerative effect, instead of the common reaction to foreign body typical of conventional hernia implants. The inherent springiness of the newly developed 3D scaffold also served to obtain a

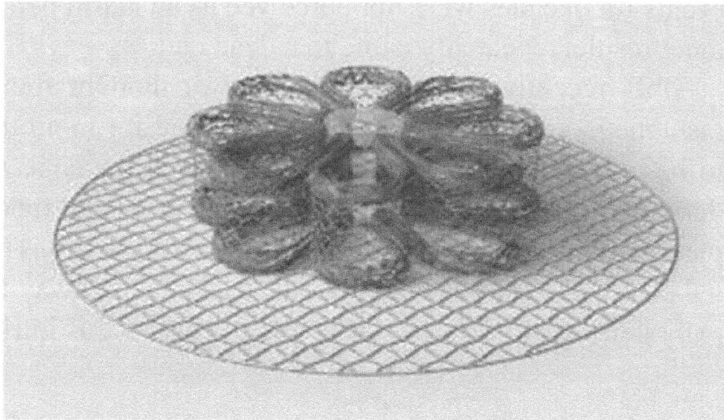

Fig. 8.2 The ProFlor 3D dynamic responsive scaffold for inguinal hernia repair

centrifugal effect which was ideal for fixation free, permanent deployment into the hernia defect. Once manufactured, this type of newly prototyped device was experimentally tested, and the working hypothesis could be confirmed as effective: a new kind of inguinal hernia device was born [25].

8.4 A New Category of Devices for a more Physiologic and Pathogenetically Coherent Treatment of Inguinal Hernia

The forerunner of this new vision has already been developed for human use following the principles of physiology of the groin and the etiology of inguinal hernia portrayed in the preceding chapters of this book. Called ProFlor, experimentally tested and clinically verified, it has been conceived as a specially designed multilamellar 3D scaffold (Fig. 8.2).

Provided with proprietary dynamic responsivity thanks to its reinforced edges, ProFlor is introduced into the hernia opening for permanent obliteration. As a result of its inherent centrifugal expansion it is positioned fully fixation free. After long years of research in the field, it can now be affirmed that ProFlor has opened a new era in the treatment of inguinal protrusions. It constitutes a completely new type of therapy model for the cure of inguinal hernia in line with the physiology of the groin and is ideal for overcoming the degenerative damage caused by inguinal protrusions [26–31]. Summarizing, embodied in this new category of hernia device there are four completely new, advanced concepts for the treatment of inguinal hernia: regenerative scaffold, dynamic responsive behavior, permanent defect obliteration, and fixation free deployment. Owing to these innovative characteristics ProFlor likely represents a turning point in the cure of inguinal hernia.

References

1. Bassini E. Sulla cura radicale dell'ernia inguinale. Arch Soc Ital di Chir. 1887;4:380.
2. Shouldice EE. The treatment of hernia. Ont Med Rev. 1953:1–14.
3. McVay CB. The anatomical bases for inguinal and femoral hernioplasty. Surg Gynecol Obstet. 1974;139:131.
4. Usher FC, Gannon JP. Marlex mesh, a new plastic mesh for replacing tissue defects. I. Experimental studies. AMA Arch Surg. 1959;78(1):131–7.
5. Lichtenstein IL, Shulman AG, Amid PK, Montllor MM. The tension-free hernioplasty. Am J Surg. 1989;157(2):188–93.
6. Lichtenstein IL, Shulman AG. Ambulatory outpatient hernia surgery. Including a new concept, introducing tension—free repair. Int Surg. 1986;71:1–4.
7. Rutkow IM, Robbins AW. The mesh-plug hernioplasty. Surg Clin North Am. 1993;73:501–12.
8. LeBlanc KA. Complications associated with the plug-and-patch method of inguinal herniorrhaphy. Hernia. 2001;5:135–8.
9. Bell RCW, Price JG. Laparoscopic inguinal hernia repair using an anatomically contoured three-dimensional mesh. Surg Endosc. 2003;17(11):1784–8.
10. Amid PK. Causes, prevention, and surgical treatment of postherniorrhaphy neuropathic inguinodynia: triple neurectomy with proximal end implantation. Hernia. 2004;8:343–9.
11. Bay-Nielsen M, Perkins FM, Kehlet H. Danish hernia database pain and functional impairment 1 year after inguinal herniorrhaphy: a nationwide questionnaire study. Am J Surg. 2001;233:1–7.
12. Bay-Nielsen M, Nilsson E, Nordin P, Kehlet H. Swedish Hernia Data Base the Danish Hernia Data Base Chronic pain after open mesh and sutured repair of indirect inguinal hernia in young males. Br J Surg. 2004;91:1372–6.
13. Kehlet H, Bay-Nielsen M. Nationwide quality improvement of groin hernia repair from the Danish Hernia Database of 87,840 patients from 1998 to 2005. Hernia. 2008;12:1–7.
14. Nienhuijs S, Staal E, Strobbe L, Rosman C, Groenewoud H. Bleichrodt R chronic pain after mesh repair of inguinal hernia: a systematic review. Am J Surg. 2007;194:394–400.
15. Loos MJ, Roumen RM, Scheltinga MR. Classifying postherniorrhaphy pain syndromes following elective inguinal hernia repair. World J Surg. 2007;31:1760–5.
16. Aasvang EK, Gmaehle E, Hansen JB, et al. Predictive risk factors for persistent postherniotomy pain. Anesthesiology. 2010;112(4):957–69.
17. Andresen K, Rosenberg J. Management of chronic pain after hernia repair. J Pain Res. 2018;11:675–81.
18. Amato G, Agrusa A, Romano G, Salamone G, Gulotta G, Silvestri F, Bussani R. Muscle degeneration in inguinal hernia specimens. Hernia. 2012;16(3):327–31.
19. Amato G, Romano G, Salamone G, Agrusa A, Saladino VA, Silvestri F, Bussani R. Damage to the vascular structures in inguinal hernia specimens. Hernia. 2012;16:63–7.
20. Amato G, Agrusa A, Romano G, Salamone G, Cocorullo G, Mularo SA, Marasa S, Gulotta G. Histological findings in direct inguinal hernia. Hernia. 2013;17(6):757–63.
21. Amato G, Agrusa A, Rodolico V, Puleio R, Di Buono G, Amodeo S, Gulotta E, Romano G. Combined inguinal hernia in the elderly. Portraying the progression of hernia disease. Int J Surg. 2016;(Suppl 1):S20-9.
22. Amato G, Calò PG, Rodolico V, Puleio R, Agrusa A, Gulotta L, Gordini L, Romano G. The septum Inguinalis: a clue to hernia genesis? J Investig Surg. 2018;31:1–9.
23. Amato G, Agrusa A, Rodolico V, Caló PG, Puleio R, Romano G. Inguinal hernia: the destiny of the inferior epigastric vessels and the pathogenesis of the disease. Surg Technol Int. 2020;18:36.
24. Amato G, Lo Monte AI, Cassata DG, Romano G, Bussani R. A new prosthetic implant for inguinal hernia repair: its features in a porcine experimental model. Artif Organs. 2011;35(8):E181–90.

25. Amato G, Romano G, Agrusa A, Marasa S, Cocorullo G, Gulotta G, Goetze T, Puleio R. Biologic response of inguinal hernia prosthetics: a comparative study of conventional static meshes versus 3D dynamic implants. Artif Organs. 2015;39(1):E10-23.
26. Amato G, Romano G, Puleio R, Agrusa A, Goetze T, Gulotta E, Gordini L, Erdas E, Calò P. Neomyogenesis in 3D dynamic responsive prosthesis for inguinal hernia repair. Artif Organs. 2018;42(12):1216–23.
27. Amato G, Agrusa A, Puleio R, Calò PG, Goetze T, Romano G. Neo-nervegenesis in 3D dynamic responsive implant for inguinal hernia repair. Qualitative study. Int J Surg. 2020;76:114–9.
28. Amato G, Agrusa A, Di Buono G, Calò PG, Casata G, Cicero L, Romano G. Inguinal hernia: defect obliteration with the 3D dynamic regenerative scaffold Proflor™. Surg Technol Int. 2021;38:199–20.
29. Amato G, Puleio R, Rodolico V, Agrusa A, Calò PG, Di Buono G, Romano G, Goetze T. Enhanced angiogenesis in the 3D dynamic responsive implant for inguinal hernia repair ProFlor®. Artif Organs. 2021:1–10.
30. Amato G, Agrusa A, Romano G. Fixation-free inguinal hernia repair using a dynamic self-retaining implant. Surg Technol Int. 2012;30:XXII. 22/17
31. Amato G, Ober E, Romano G, Salamone G, Agrusa A, Gulotta G, Bussani R. Nerve degeneration in inguinal hernia specimens. Hernia. 2011;15:53–8.

[illegible]

[illegible] 2011). DALYs and dis- [illegible] because NCDs are [illegible] public health strategy, and the presence of supportive [illegible] and environmental factors for NCDs may become more prominent [illegible] from healthcare services (Flynn and Cooper 2019). The need for attention to clinical care and public health policies has resulted in the survival of patients, who may have been lost to infections, malnutrition, and [illegible] suggests increasing DALYs (disability-associated life years) [illegible]

4.5 Challenges Faced by Low- and Middle-Income Countries

[illegible]

GPSR Compliance

The European Union's (EU) General Product Safety Regulation (GPSR) is a set of rules that requires consumer products to be safe and our obligations to ensure this.

If you have any concerns about our products, you can contact us on ProductSafety@springernature.com

In case Publisher is established outside the EU, the EU authorized representative is:

Springer Nature Customer Service Center GmbH
Europaplatz 3
69115 Heidelberg, Germany

Batch number: 10739787

Printed by Printforce, the Netherlands